# Contents

- **Preface**
- **Chapters**
- **Conclusion**
- **References**
- **Index**
- **Author's Profile**

# Preface

The quest to understand the human body, to alleviate suffering, and to extend the reach of life itself is a story as old as humanity. Throughout history, individuals have emerged—driven by curiosity, compassion, and a relentless pursuit of knowledge—to transform the art and science of healing. This book, **"Trailblazers in Healing:** A Global History of Medicine Through 100 Remarkable Lives," is a tribute to those who have left an enduring mark on the field we call medicine.

Within these pages, we embark on a journey across time and cultures, exploring the lives of 100 individuals who have shaped the course of medical history. From the ancient wisdom of Hippocrates to the groundbreaking surgeries of the 20th century, and the revolutionary scientific discoveries of our modern era, each chapter offers a glimpse into the brilliance, perseverance, and sometimes the struggles of these medical pioneers.

This is not merely a recounting of names and dates. It is an exploration of the human stories behind the medical breakthroughs—the moments of inspiration, the challenges overcome, the ethical dilemmas faced, and the legacies that continue to shape healthcare today. We will travel from the bustling hospitals of ancient Alexandria to the serene gardens where Chinese herbalists discovered potent remedies, and from the laboratories where scientists unlocked the secrets of DNA to the operating rooms where surgeons dared to attempt the impossible.

**"Trailblazers in Healing"** embraces a global perspective, recognizing that medical knowledge has always been a tapestry woven from the contributions of diverse cultures and traditions. We will meet not only those whose names are etched in Western medical textbooks but also individuals from Egypt, India, China, Africa, and the Islamic world who have enriched the global understanding of healing.

As you delve into these remarkable lives, I invite you to reflect on the enduring themes that connect them: the power of observation, the drive for innovation, the importance of collaboration, and above all, the profound sense of compassion that lies at the heart of medicine. May their stories inspire a new generation of healers, scientists, and advocates to continue the quest for knowledge and to carry the torch of medical progress forward.

Sincerely,

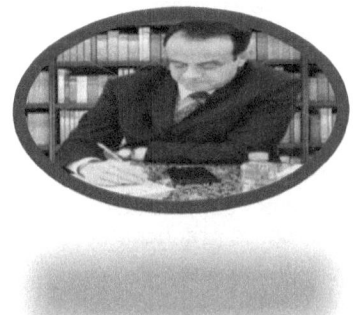

Dr. Atef Ahmed

[2024]

books.dratef.net
dratef1980@gmail.com

1. **Hippocrates (Ancient Greece): The Father of Medicine**
    - Opening Quote: "Life is short, and Art long; the occasion fleeting; experience fallacious, and judgment difficult." – Hippocrates
    - Historical Context: Ancient Greece, a time of philosophical and scientific inquiry, but also reliance on supernatural explanations for illness.
    - Early Life & Influences: Born on the island of Kos, family background in the Asclepiad tradition (healers), likely studied at the temple of Asclepius.
    - Major Contributions:
        - The Hippocratic Corpus: Collection of medical texts, emphasis on observation, diagnosis based on symptoms, natural explanations for disease.
        - The Hippocratic Oath: Foundation of medical ethics, "First, do no harm," patient confidentiality, acting in the best interest of the patient.
    - Challenges & Controversies: Debate over the authorship of the Hippocratic Corpus, some practices based on the Four Humors theory now debunked.
    - Global Impact & Legacy:
        - Foundation of Western medical ethics.
        - The shift from supernatural to natural explanations for illness.
        - Importance of observation and clinical diagnosis, a lasting influence on medical education.
    - "Beyond the Scalpel": Some accounts suggest Hippocrates traveled extensively, treating patients in various Greek cities, demonstrating a commitment to serving humanity.
2. **Sushruta (Ancient India): The Father of Surgery**
    - Opening Quote: "Surgery is the first and the highest division of the healing art, pure in itself, perpetual in its applicability, a working field for the courageous, and a source of fame." – Sushruta Samhita
    - Historical Context: Ancient India, a time of advanced philosophical thought and a holistic approach to medicine (Ayurveda).
    - Early Life & Influences: Little known about his life, but his teachings are preserved in the Sushruta Samhita, a surgical treatise.
    - Major Contributions:
        - Sushruta Samhita: Detailed surgical techniques, over 300 surgical procedures described, 121 surgical instruments, plastic surgery (rhinoplasty).

- o Emphasis on anatomy: Believed understanding anatomy was essential for surgical skill.
- o Ethical guidelines for surgeons: Compassionate care, lifelong learning, and professional conduct.
- Challenges & Controversies: Some surgical techniques, like bloodletting, are no longer practiced.
- Global Impact & Legacy:
  - o Influential on the development of surgery in India and beyond.
  - o Early recognition of the importance of specialized surgical training.
  - o Legacy seen in modern plastic surgery techniques.
- "Beyond the Scalpel": The Sushruta Samhita emphasizes the importance of a surgeon's character, stating that surgical skill should be coupled with compassion and ethical conduct.

## 3. Zhang Zhongjing (Ancient China): The Sage of Traditional Chinese Medicine

- Opening Quote: "To cure disease, one must first know its root cause." – Zhang Zhongjing
- Historical Context: Han Dynasty in China, development of codified medical knowledge within Traditional Chinese Medicine.
- Early Life & Influences: Served as a government official and physician, witnessed widespread suffering during epidemics, which inspired his medical work.
- Major Contributions:
  - o Shang Han Lun (Treatise on Cold Damage Diseases): Detailed clinical descriptions of diseases and their symptoms, emphasis on pattern identification and differentiation.
  - o Foundation of Chinese herbal medicine: Detailed formulas and prescriptions using combinations of herbs to restore balance and harmony.
- Challenges & Controversies: TCM theories differ significantly from Western medicine, which can create challenges for integration.
- Global Impact & Legacy:
  - o Fundamental text of TCM, still studied and practiced today.
  - o Influenced the development of herbal medicine throughout East Asia.
  - o Growing interest in TCM worldwide as a complementary approach to healthcare.
- "Beyond the Scalpel": Zhang Zhongjing's work shows a deep understanding of human physiology and a compassionate approach to treating the sick.

## 4. Agnodice (Ancient Greece): A Pioneer Woman in Medicine

- Opening Quote: "For the love of healing, I disguised myself." – Attributed to Agnodice
- Historical Context: Ancient Greece, a time when women were excluded from most professions, including medicine.

- Early Life & Influences: According to legend, Agnodice disguised herself as a man to study medicine and practice as a physician in Athens.
- Major Contributions:
  - Defied societal norms: Her story highlights the barriers women faced in entering the medical profession.
  - Specialized in women's health: Provided care to women who were reluctant to be examined by male physicians.
- Challenges & Controversies: Her story is likely a legend, but it highlights the exclusion of women from medicine in ancient times.
- Global Impact & Legacy:
  - A symbolic figure for women's fight for equality in healthcare.
  - Represents the importance of access to female physicians for women's health.
- "Beyond the Scalpel": Agnodice's story, whether fact or fiction, has inspired generations of women to pursue careers in medicine.

## 5. Pedanius Dioscorides (Ancient Rome): The Father of Pharmacology

- Opening Quote: "Nature is the best physician." – Attributed to Dioscorides
- Historical Context: Roman Empire, a time of expanding knowledge about the natural world and medicinal plants.
- Early Life & Influences: Served as a physician in the Roman army, traveled extensively, collecting knowledge about medicinal plants.
- Major Contributions:
  - De Materia Medica: A five-volume encyclopedia of medicinal plants, described over 600 plants, their properties, and uses.
  - Influential on the development of pharmacology: His work remained a standard reference for centuries.
- Challenges & Controversies: Some of his remedies are now considered ineffective or even harmful.
- Global Impact & Legacy:
  - De Materia Medica was translated into many languages and used throughout the Middle Ages and Renaissance.
  - Foundation of pharmacognosy (the study of natural drugs).
  - Influence on modern herbal medicine and the search for new drug compounds.
- "Beyond the Scalpel": Dioscorides' work shows a deep appreciation for the healing power of nature.

## 6. Galen (Ancient Rome): Anatomist and Physician of the Roman Empire

- Opening Quote: "The best physician is also a philosopher." – Galen
- Historical Context: Roman Empire, a time of relative peace and prosperity, allowing for advancements in science and medicine.
- Early Life & Influences: Born in Pergamon (now Turkey), studied medicine in Alexandria (Egypt), a center of medical knowledge.
- Major Contributions:

- o  Prolific writer on medicine: His works were influential for over 1,500 years.
- o  Detailed anatomical studies: Dissections of animals (human dissection was forbidden), provided insights into the human body.
- o  Theory of the four humors: Influenced medical practice for centuries (though later debunked).
* Challenges & Controversies: His anatomical studies had inaccuracies due to the reliance on animal dissection.
* Global Impact & Legacy:
  - o  His work was the basis of medical education in Europe for centuries.
  - o  His emphasis on understanding physiology influenced the development of medical science.
* "Beyond the Scalpel": Galen's confidence in his own abilities was legendary; he often publicly challenged other physicians, demonstrating his strong personality.

## 7. Al-Razi (Rhazes) (Persia): The Clinician and Empiricist

* Opening Quote: "The physician must be an investigator." – Al-Razi
* Historical Context: Islamic Golden Age, a time of flourishing intellectual and scientific advancements.
* Early Life & Influences: Born in Ray, Persia (now Iran), head physician at a Baghdad hospital, known for his clinical skills and observational powers.
* Major Contributions:
  - o  Al-Hawi (The Comprehensive Book): A vast medical encyclopedia compiling his own observations and the knowledge of Greek, Indian, and Persian physicians.
  - o  Differentiated smallpox from measles: Detailed clinical descriptions, a significant contribution to epidemiology.
  - o  Advocated for experimentation and clinical trials: A pioneer of empirical medicine.
* Challenges & Controversies: Some of his treatments are considered outdated by modern standards.
* Global Impact & Legacy:
  - o  Al-Hawi was a standard medical text in Europe for centuries.
  - o  His emphasis on clinical observation and experimentation influenced the development of medical science.
* "Beyond the Scalpel": Al-Razi was known for his compassion for the poor and his commitment to providing free medical care.

## 8. Avicenna (Ibn Sina) (Persia): The Polymath Physician

* Opening Quote: "Medicine is a science by which we learn the various states of the human body, in health, when not in health, the means by which health is likely to be lost, and, when lost, is likely to be restored." – Avicenna
* Historical Context: Islamic Golden Age, a time of intellectual and scientific flourishing.

- Early Life & Influences: A prodigious intellect, memorized the Quran by age 10, studied philosophy, mathematics, and medicine.
- Major Contributions:
    - The Canon of Medicine: A vast and influential medical encyclopedia that synthesized medical knowledge, organized it logically, and added new insights.
    - Covered a wide range of topics: Anatomy, physiology, hygiene, diagnosis, treatment, pharmacology, and surgery.
    - Introduced new ideas: Quarantine for contagious diseases, the concept of clinical trials.
- Challenges & Controversies: Some of his medical theories, based on the prevailing knowledge of the time, are now outdated.
- Global Impact & Legacy:
    - The Canon of Medicine became a standard text in both Islamic and European medical schools for centuries.
    - His work bridged the gap between ancient and modern medicine, laying the groundwork for a more systematic and scientific approach.
- "Beyond the Scalpel": Avicenna was a prolific writer in many fields, including philosophy, poetry, astronomy, and music, demonstrating his extraordinary intellect.

## 9. Trotula of Salerno (Italy): A Medieval Woman Physician

- Opening Quote: "Women should not be ashamed to speak of their problems." – Attributed to Trotula
- Historical Context: 11th-century Salerno, Italy, a center of medical learning where the Schola Medica Salernitana, a medical school open to women, flourished.
- Early Life & Influences: Little is known about her life, but she is believed to have been a physician and teacher at the Schola Medica Salernitana.
- Major Contributions:
    - Writings on women's health: Authorship debated, but the Trotula, a collection of texts on women's medicine, was attributed to her.
    - Topics included: Gynecology, obstetrics, cosmetics, and infertility.
    - Offered practical advice: On childbirth, menstrual problems, and skin care.
- Challenges & Controversies: Authorship of the Trotula is debated, but her existence as a female physician at Salerno is generally accepted.
- Global Impact & Legacy:
    - The Trotula was widely circulated in Europe and influential in women's medicine.
    - Her work, regardless of exact authorship, represents the vital role of women in healthcare throughout history.
- "Beyond the Scalpel": Trotula's work challenged the societal norms of the time, which often excluded women from medicine.

## 10. Ibn al-Nafis (Syria): Discoverer of Pulmonary Circulation

- Opening Quote: "Blood must arrive at the right cavity of the heart, but there is no direct pathway between them." – Ibn al-Nafis
- Historical Context: Islamic Golden Age, a time of flourishing scientific inquiry, especially in anatomy and physiology.
- Early Life & Influences: Born in Damascus, Syria, studied medicine, served as a physician at a Cairo hospital, known for his meticulous anatomical studies.
- Major Contributions:
    - Commentary on Anatomy in Avicenna's Canon: Corrected Galen's errors in anatomy, first to accurately describe pulmonary circulation (blood flow from the heart to the lungs).
- Challenges & Controversies: His work was not known in Europe until the 20th century, so credit for the discovery of pulmonary circulation was initially given to European scientists.
- Global Impact & Legacy:
    - A vital contribution to the understanding of the cardiovascular system.
    - Demonstrates the advancements made in Islamic medicine during the Golden Age.
- "Beyond the Scalpel": Ibn al-Nafis was also a scholar of Islamic law and jurisprudence, demonstrating his wide-ranging intellectual interests.

## 11. Hildegard von Bingen (Germany): A Medieval Abbess and Healer

- Opening Quote: "The soul must be healed along with the body." – Hildegard von Bingen
- Historical Context: 12th-century Germany, a time of great religious devotion and monastic life.
- Early Life & Influences: A Benedictine abbess, visionary, composer, and writer. She experienced mystical visions and believed in the interconnectedness of the body and spirit.
- Major Contributions:
    - Physica and Causae et Curae: Writings on natural history and medicine, combining religious beliefs with practical knowledge of herbs and remedies.
    - Holistic approach to healing: Emphasized diet, exercise, music, and spiritual practices for well-being.
- Challenges & Controversies: Her medical practices were rooted in religious beliefs, which are not always aligned with modern medical science.
- Global Impact & Legacy:
    - Her writings provide insights into medieval medicine and the role of women in healing.
    - Renewed interest in her holistic approach to health and the integration of spirituality and medicine.

- "Beyond the Scalpel": Hildegard von Bingen was a remarkable polymath, a composer, poet, and playwright, demonstrating a wide-ranging intellect and artistic talent.

## 12. Andreas Vesalius (Flanders): Revolutionizing Anatomy

- Opening Quote: "I am not accustomed to saying anything with certainty after only one or two observations." – Andreas Vesalius
- Historical Context: Renaissance, a time of rediscovering classical knowledge and challenging established authority.
- Early Life & Influences: Studied medicine in Paris, but frustrated with traditional teaching based on Galen, he began his own dissections.
- Major Contributions:
    - De Humani Corporis Fabrica (On the Fabric of the Human Body): A landmark anatomical text with detailed illustrations based on his own dissections, corrected many of Galen's errors.
- Challenges & Controversies: Challenging Galen's authority was risky, and he faced criticism from traditionalists.
- Global Impact & Legacy:
    - Transformed the study of anatomy, moving it from textual reliance to direct observation.
    - His work laid the foundation for modern anatomical science.
- "Beyond the Scalpel": Vesalius' beautiful anatomical illustrations, often in dramatic poses, are considered works of art in their own right.

## 13. Ambroise Paré (France): The Father of Modern Surgery

- Opening Quote: "I dressed him, God healed him." - Ambroise Paré
- Historical Context: Renaissance, warfare leading to advances in battlefield surgery.
- Early Life & Influences: Began as a barber-surgeon, served in the French army, witnessing firsthand the brutality of battlefield wounds.
- Major Contributions:
    - Rejected cauterization of wounds: Introduced gentler methods of treating gunshot wounds using ligatures (tying off blood vessels) instead of hot irons.
    - Improved prosthetics: Designed more functional artificial limbs.
- Challenges & Controversies: Faced resistance from traditional surgeons who clung to older methods.
- Global Impact & Legacy:
    - His innovations led to a more humane approach to surgery.
    - Considered a founder of modern surgical practice.
- "Beyond the Scalpel": Paré was known for his compassion and his belief that surgery should be a last resort, always seeking less invasive methods whenever possible.

## 14. William Harvey (England): Discoverer of Blood Circulation

- Opening Quote: "Let us go back to the heart, the supreme organ." - William Harvey
- Historical Context: Scientific Revolution, increasing reliance on experimentation and observation.
- Early Life & Influences: Studied at the University of Padua, influenced by the work of anatomists like Fabricius.
- Major Contributions:
    - De Motu Cordis (On the Motion of the Heart and Blood): Detailed his experiments and observations, proving that blood circulates throughout the body, pumped by the heart.
- Challenges & Controversies: His theory challenged Galen's idea that blood was constantly being produced and consumed, initially met with resistance.
- Global Impact & Legacy:
    - Fundamental to our understanding of physiology and the cardiovascular system.
    - His work marked a shift toward a more scientific approach to understanding the body.
- "Beyond the Scalpel": Harvey was also a physician to King James I and King Charles I of England, demonstrating his high standing in the medical community.

### 15. Paracelsus (Switzerland): The Alchemist Physician
- Opening Quote: "The dose makes the poison." – Paracelsus
- Historical Context: Renaissance, a time of transition in alchemy and medicine.
- Early Life & Influences: Swiss physician, alchemist, and philosopher. Rejected traditional medical teachings and emphasized the use of chemicals and minerals in medicine.
- Major Contributions:
    - Pioneer of chemical pharmacology: Introduced the use of mercury to treat syphilis.
    - Challenged traditional medical authority: Argued for observation and experimentation, rather than relying on ancient texts.
- Challenges & Controversies: His unorthodox methods and abrasive personality brought him many enemies.
- Global Impact & Legacy:
    - Influence on the development of pharmacology and the use of chemicals in medicine.
    - His holistic view of illness considered a precursor to mind-body medicine.
- "Beyond the Scalpel": Paracelsus was known for his eccentricities and his belief in the power of nature to heal.

### 16. Edward Jenner (England): The Pioneer of Vaccination
- Opening Quote: "The annihilation of the smallpox, the most dreadful scourge of the human species, must be the final result of this practice." – Edward Jenner

- Historical Context: 18th century, smallpox was a deadly and widespread disease.
- Early Life & Influences: Country physician, observed that milkmaids who contracted cowpox seemed immune to smallpox.
- Major Contributions:
    - Developed the first smallpox vaccine: Inoculated a boy with cowpox, proving that it provided immunity against smallpox.
- Challenges & Controversies: Vaccination was initially met with fear and resistance from some who considered it unnatural or dangerous.
- Global Impact & Legacy:
    - Led to the worldwide eradication of smallpox.
    - Laid the foundation for modern immunology and vaccination programs, saving millions of lives.
- "Beyond the Scalpel": Jenner was a keen naturalist and observer, fascinated by the natural world.

## 17. James Parkinson (England): Identifying Parkinson's Disease

- Opening Quote: "Involuntary tremulous motion, with lessened muscular power, in parts not in action and even when supported; with a propensity to bend the trunk forwards, and to pass from a walking to a running pace: the senses and intellects being uninjured." – James Parkinson describing the symptoms of the disease that would later bear his name.
- Historical Context: Early 19th century, little understanding of neurological disorders.
- Early Life & Influences: English surgeon, apothecary, and paleontologist, interested in a wide range of scientific pursuits.
- Major Contributions:
    - An Essay on the Shaking Palsy: Described six cases of the disease, detailing the distinctive symptoms, later named Parkinson's disease.
- Challenges & Controversies: His work was largely ignored during his lifetime, and recognition for his discovery came much later.
- Global Impact & Legacy:
    - His meticulous observations laid the foundation for research on Parkinson's disease.
    - His work is essential to the ongoing efforts to understand and treat this debilitating condition.
- "Beyond the Scalpel": Parkinson was also a social activist, involved in reform movements and concerned about the welfare of the poor.

## 18. René Laennec (France): The Inventor of the Stethoscope

- Opening Quote: "I was struck with the idea of employing... a cylinder of wood." – René Laennec on the inspiration for the stethoscope.
- Historical Context: Early 19th century, diagnosis relied heavily on observation and palpation, difficult to hear internal sounds clearly.
- Early Life & Influences: French physician, particularly interested in diseases of the chest (tuberculosis was rampant).

- Major Contributions:
  - Invented the stethoscope: Inspired by watching children transmitting sound through wooden planks, he created a wooden cylinder that amplified sounds from the chest.
- Challenges & Controversies: Initially, some physicians were skeptical of the new instrument.
- Global Impact & Legacy:
  - The stethoscope revolutionized medical diagnosis, allowing physicians to hear heart and lung sounds clearly.
  - It remains an iconic symbol of the medical profession and is an essential tool for diagnosis.
- "Beyond the Scalpel": Laennec was known for his meticulous clinical observations and his dedication to improving the understanding of chest diseases.

### 19. Ignaz Semmelweis (Hungary): The Savior of Mothers

- Opening Quote: "To combat puerperal fever, handwashing is imperative!" - Ignaz Semmelweis
- Historical Context: Mid-19th century, childbirth was a dangerous event due to high rates of puerperal fever (childbed fever).
- Early Life & Influences: Hungarian physician, appalled by the high mortality rate of women in childbirth at the Vienna General Hospital.
- Major Contributions:
  - Discovered the link between hand hygiene and puerperal fever: Observed that medical students carrying "cadaveric particles" from autopsies were infecting mothers.
  - Implemented handwashing with chlorinated lime: This drastically reduced puerperal fever rates.
- Challenges & Controversies: Faced strong resistance from colleagues who refused to accept his findings, his ideas were not widely adopted until after his death.
- Global Impact & Legacy:
  - A pioneer of infection control.
  - His work laid the foundation for modern antiseptic practices, saving countless lives.
- "Beyond the Scalpel": Semmelweis' tragic story highlights the importance of challenging medical dogma and the need for evidence-based practice.

### 20. Florence Nightingale (England): The Founder of Modern Nursing

- Opening Quote: "I think one's feelings waste themselves in words; they ought all to be distilled into actions which bring results." - Florence Nightingale
- Historical Context: 19th century, nursing was considered a menial task, hospitals lacked hygiene standards.
- Early Life & Influences: Born into a wealthy family, defied societal expectations to pursue a career in nursing, inspired by a religious calling to serve others.

- Major Contributions:
    - Transformed nursing during the Crimean War: Improved sanitary conditions, implemented systematic care, reduced mortality rates.
    - Established professional nursing schools: Founded the Nightingale Training School, emphasizing education and high standards of care.
- Challenges & Controversies: Faced initial resistance from military officials, later struggled with illness that limited her activities.
- Global Impact & Legacy:
    - Elevated nursing to a respected profession.
    - Her emphasis on hygiene, sanitation, and patient-centered care revolutionized hospitals and healthcare.
- "Beyond the Scalpel": Nightingale was a gifted writer and statistician, using data to advocate for healthcare reforms and improvements.

## 21. Elizabeth Blackwell (USA): The First Woman Doctor in the U.S.

- Opening Quote: "It is not easy to be a pioneer – but oh, it is fascinating! I would not trade one moment, even the worst moment, for all the riches in the world." – Elizabeth Blackwell
- Historical Context: 19th century USA, women were largely excluded from higher education and the medical profession.
- Early Life & Influences: Inspired to become a doctor after a friend's death, faced constant rejection from medical schools due to her gender.
- Major Contributions:
    - Became the first woman to graduate from medical school in the USA (Geneva Medical College, 1849).
    - Founded the New York Infirmary for Women and Children: Providing healthcare to underserved women and training female physicians.
- Challenges & Controversies: Faced prejudice and discrimination throughout her career, struggled to gain acceptance in the male-dominated medical world.
- Global Impact & Legacy:
    - A pioneer for women in medicine, opening doors for future generations of female physicians.
    - Her work emphasized the importance of social reform and public health.
- "Beyond the Scalpel": Blackwell was a strong advocate for women's rights and social justice, challenging societal norms and campaigning for women's suffrage.

## 22. Louis Pasteur (France): The Father of Microbiology

- Opening Quote: "Science knows no country, because knowledge belongs to humanity, and is the torch which illuminates the world." – Louis Pasteur
- Historical Context: 19th century, a time of scientific ferment and the emergence of the germ theory of disease.

- Early Life & Influences: French chemist and microbiologist, originally focused on crystallography, but his research on fermentation led him to the world of microbes.
- Major Contributions:
  - Developed germ theory: Proved that microorganisms were responsible for fermentation and disease, debunking the theory of spontaneous generation.
  - Invented pasteurization: A process of heating to kill harmful bacteria in liquids, revolutionized food safety.
  - Developed vaccines for rabies, anthrax, and chicken cholera: Demonstrating the power of immunization to prevent disease.
- Challenges & Controversies: Faced skepticism and resistance from some scientists, had to defend his theories through rigorous experimentation.
- Global Impact & Legacy:
  - His discoveries transformed medicine and public health, leading to the development of antibiotics, vaccines, and sterilization techniques.
  - His work saved countless lives and continues to inspire research in infectious diseases.
- "Beyond the Scalpel": Pasteur was a passionate patriot, deeply affected by the Franco-Prussian War and determined to use science to improve the lives of his countrymen.

## 23. Robert Koch (Germany): The Father of Bacteriology

- Opening Quote: "Every disease has its specific germ." - Robert Koch
- Historical Context: 19th century, the golden age of bacteriology, following Pasteur's work on germ theory.
- Early Life & Influences: German physician, fascinated by the world of microorganisms, inspired by Pasteur's research.
- Major Contributions:
  - Identified the bacteria responsible for anthrax, tuberculosis, and cholera: Developed techniques to isolate and study bacteria in pure cultures.
  - Koch's Postulates: Established criteria to link a specific microorganism to a specific disease, fundamental to modern microbiology.
- Challenges & Controversies: His tuberculin, a proposed treatment for tuberculosis, proved ineffective and caused controversy.
- Global Impact & Legacy:
  - His discoveries were essential to understanding and controlling major infectious diseases.
  - His work laid the foundation for modern bacteriology and public health measures to prevent the spread of disease.
- "Beyond the Scalpel": Koch was a dedicated researcher, working tirelessly in his laboratory to unlock the secrets of infectious diseases.

## 24. Joseph Lister (England): The Pioneer of Antiseptic Surgery

- Opening Quote: "It is the duty of the surgeon to eliminate sepsis." – Joseph Lister
- Historical Context: 19th century, surgery was extremely dangerous due to high rates of postoperative infection.
- Early Life & Influences: British surgeon, deeply influenced by Pasteur's germ theory of disease.
- Major Contributions:
  - Introduced antiseptic techniques in surgery: Used carbolic acid (phenol) to sterilize instruments, dressings, and the operating room.
- Challenges & Controversies: Faced resistance from traditional surgeons who were reluctant to abandon old practices.
- Global Impact & Legacy:
  - Lister's methods dramatically reduced surgical mortality rates.
  - His work revolutionized surgery, making it a safer and more effective treatment option.
- "Beyond the Scalpel": Lister was a Quaker, and his religious beliefs influenced his deep concern for the well-being of his patients.

### 25. Marie Curie (Poland/France): The Pioneer of Radioactivity

- Opening Quote: "Nothing in life is to be feared, it is only to be understood. Now is the time to understand more, so that we may fear less." – Marie Curie
- Historical Context: Late 19th and early 20th centuries, a time of rapid advancements in physics and chemistry.
- Early Life & Influences: Born Maria Skłodowska in Poland, faced discrimination as a woman in science, studied in Paris, met Pierre Curie, her collaborator and husband.
- Major Contributions:
  - Pioneered research on radioactivity: Discovered polonium and radium, two new radioactive elements.
  - Developed techniques to isolate radioactive isotopes: Laid the foundation for nuclear medicine.
- Challenges & Controversies: The dangers of radiation were not fully understood, and she suffered health problems due to prolonged exposure.
- Global Impact & Legacy:
  - Her work revolutionized our understanding of atomic structure.
  - Her discoveries led to the development of radiation therapy for cancer and other medical applications of radioactivity.
- "Beyond the Scalpel": Marie Curie was the first woman to win a Nobel Prize and the only person to win Nobel Prizes in two different scientific fields (Physics and Chemistry).

### 26. Sigmund Freud (Austria): The Father of Psychoanalysis

- Opening Quote: "Unexpressed emotions will never die. They are buried alive and will come forth later in uglier ways." – Sigmund Freud

- Historical Context: Late 19th and early 20th centuries, a time of exploring the human mind and the emergence of psychology.
- Early Life & Influences: Austrian neurologist, frustrated with the limitations of neurology, sought new ways to understand and treat mental illness.
- Major Contributions:
  - Developed psychoanalysis: A theory of the mind that emphasized the unconscious, dream interpretation, and the influence of childhood experiences on adult behavior.
  - Introduced new concepts: The id, ego, and superego, defense mechanisms, and psychosexual stages of development.
- Challenges & Controversies: Many of his theories were considered radical and controversial, psychoanalysis has been both praised and criticized.
- Global Impact & Legacy:
  - His work had a profound impact on psychology, psychiatry, and even culture, changing the way we view the human mind.
  - His ideas continue to be debated and explored.
- "Beyond the Scalpel": Freud was a prolific writer and a keen observer of human behavior, drawing inspiration from literature, art, and mythology.

## 27. Alexander Fleming (Scotland): The Discoverer of Penicillin

- Opening Quote: "One sometimes finds what one is not looking for." – Alexander Fleming
- Historical Context: Early 20th century, bacterial infections were a major cause of death, no effective treatments available.
- Early Life & Influences: Scottish bacteriologist, known for his meticulous laboratory work and his interest in finding new ways to combat infections.
- Major Contributions:
  - Discovered penicillin: In 1928, he observed that a mold (Penicillium notatum) had killed bacteria in a petri dish, leading to the development of the first antibiotic.
- Challenges & Controversies: Initially, it was difficult to produce penicillin in large quantities.
- Global Impact & Legacy:
  - Penicillin revolutionized medicine, saving countless lives from bacterial infections.
  - His discovery marked the beginning of the antibiotic era, but also raised concerns about antibiotic resistance.
- "Beyond the Scalpel": Fleming was a modest and unassuming man, who never fully grasped the impact his discovery would have on the world.

## 28. Frederick Banting (Canada): The Co-Discoverer of Insulin

- Opening Quote: "Insulin does not cure diabetes; it merely controls it." – Frederick Banting

- Historical Context: Early 20th century, diabetes was a fatal disease.
- Early Life & Influences: Canadian physician, deeply moved by the suffering of diabetic patients, particularly children.
- Major Contributions:
  - Discovered insulin: With Charles Best, he isolated insulin from the pancreas of dogs, paving the way for its use in treating diabetes.
- Challenges & Controversies: The initial production of insulin was difficult, and there were disputes over credit for the discovery.
- Global Impact & Legacy:
  - Insulin transformed diabetes from a death sentence to a manageable condition.
  - His work led to advances in endocrinology and the treatment of hormonal disorders.
- "Beyond the Scalpel": Banting was a talented artist and enjoyed painting, a passion that provided a balance to his intense scientific work.

### 29. Virginia Apgar (USA): The Innovator in Neonatal Care
- Opening Quote: "Nobody, but nobody, is going to stop breathing on me!" – Virginia Apgar
- Historical Context: Mid-20th century, little attention was given to the immediate assessment of newborn health.
- Early Life & Influences: American physician, specialized in anesthesiology, concerned about the high mortality rate of newborns.
- Major Contributions:
  - Developed the Apgar score: A simple and effective method for evaluating the health of newborns, assessed five key criteria, still widely used today.
- Challenges & Controversies: Faced gender discrimination in the male-dominated field of medicine.
- Global Impact & Legacy:
  - Her work revolutionized neonatal care, leading to the prompt identification and treatment of newborns in distress, saving countless lives.
  - Her score is a testament to the importance of observation and quick assessment in medical practice.
- "Beyond the Scalpel": Apgar was a talented musician who played several instruments, and she even built her own cello.

### 30. Jonas Salk (USA): The Conqueror of Polio
- Opening Quote: "Hope lies in dreams, in imagination, and in the courage of those who dare to make dreams into reality." – Jonas Salk
- Historical Context: Mid-20th century, polio epidemics caused widespread fear and paralysis, particularly affecting children.
- Early Life & Influences: American medical researcher and virologist, driven by the desire to find a way to prevent polio.
- Major Contributions:

- o Developed the first effective polio vaccine: Used a killed-virus vaccine, a major breakthrough in the fight against polio.
- Challenges & Controversies: There were initial concerns about the safety of the inactivated polio vaccine (IPV), though it was proven effective.
- Global Impact & Legacy:
  - o Led to the dramatic decline of polio cases worldwide, polio is now close to eradication.
  - o His work demonstrated the power of vaccination to eliminate a major infectious disease.
- "Beyond the Scalpel": Salk refused to patent the polio vaccine, believing that it should be available to all children, putting public health before personal profit.

### 31. Helen Brooke Taussig (USA): Pioneer of Pediatric Cardiology
- Opening Quote: "I couldn't change what was wrong with them, but maybe I could change what happened because of it." - Helen Brooke Taussig
- Historical Context: Mid-20th century, limited understanding and treatment options for congenital heart defects in children.
- Early Life & Influences: American cardiologist, overcame dyslexia and hearing loss to excel in medicine, dedicated to helping "blue babies" (children with cyanotic heart disease).
- Major Contributions:
  - o Pioneered research on congenital heart defects: Described Tetralogy of Fallot, a complex heart defect causing "blue baby syndrome."
  - o Collaborated with Alfred Blalock and Vivien Thomas: To develop the Blalock-Taussig shunt, a surgical procedure to improve blood flow in blue babies.
- Challenges & Controversies: Faced challenges as a woman in a male-dominated field of medicine, initially met with resistance to her ideas.
- Global Impact & Legacy:
  - o Transformed the field of pediatric cardiology, her work saved the lives of countless children with heart defects.
  - o A pioneer for women in medicine.
- "Beyond the Scalpel": Taussig was a passionate advocate for children with disabilities, working to improve their access to education and care.

### 32. Christiaan Barnard (South Africa): The Heart Transplant Pioneer
- Opening Quote: "On the operating table, we are technicians. But in the recovery room, we become human again." – Christiaan Barnard
- Historical Context: 20th century, the rise of advanced surgical techniques and organ transplantation.

- Early Life & Influences: South African cardiac surgeon, trained in the USA, fascinated by the possibility of heart transplantation.
- Major Contributions:
  - Performed the first successful human-to-human heart transplant: On December 3, 1967, in Cape Town, South Africa.
- Defining Death: The criteria for determining brain death, necessary for organ donation, were not yet standardized, raising complex issues.
- Organ Allocation: The scarcity of donor organs and the criteria for deciding who receives a transplant ignited debates about fairness and resource allocation.
- Playing God?: Some critics questioned whether humans had the right to intervene in such a fundamental way with life and death, challenging the very essence of mortality.
- The Burden of Life: The long-term physical and psychological impact on transplant recipients and their families was unknown, raising concerns about quality of life and the challenges of adaptation.

## 33. Norman Shumway (USA): Pioneering Heart-Lung Transplantation

- Opening Quote: "The only limitations to heart transplantation are the limits of human imagination and creativity." – Norman Shumway
- Historical Context: 20th century, the era of exploring organ transplantation as a treatment for end-stage organ failure.
- Early Life & Influences: American surgeon, a pioneer in the development of heart-lung transplantation, dedicated to research and innovation.
- Major Contributions:
  - Perfected the technique of heart-lung transplantation: Performed the first successful adult human heart-lung transplant in 1981.
- Challenges & Controversies: Early transplants faced high risks of rejection and infection, ethical concerns about resource allocation and patient selection.
- Global Impact & Legacy:
  - His work advanced the field of transplantation and opened new possibilities for treating patients with heart and lung diseases.
  - His legacy continues to inspire research in transplant immunology and organ preservation.
- "Beyond the Scalpel": Shumway was a passionate advocate for organ donation, recognizing its life-saving potential.

## 34. Tu Youyou (China): Discoverer of Artemisinin for Malaria

- Opening Quote: "Every scientist dreams of doing something that can help the world." - Tu Youyou
- Historical Context: 20th century, malaria was a major global health threat, drug resistance was increasing.

- Early Life & Influences: Chinese pharmaceutical chemist, trained in both Western and traditional Chinese medicine, inspired by ancient texts to search for new antimalarial drugs.
- Major Contributions:
  - Discovered artemisinin: Isolated from the sweet wormwood plant (Artemisia annua), a traditional Chinese remedy, a highly effective antimalarial drug.
- Challenges & Controversies: Working during the Cultural Revolution in China posed significant obstacles to her research.
- Global Impact & Legacy:
  - Artemisinin-based combination therapies (ACTs) have become the standard treatment for malaria, saving millions of lives.
  - Her discovery highlights the importance of traditional medicine in finding new drug treatments.
- "Beyond the Scalpel": Tu Youyou's dedication to her research, even in the face of political turmoil, demonstrates her commitment to fighting a devastating disease.

## 35. David Ho (Taiwan/USA): Pioneer of HIV/AIDS Research

- Opening Quote: "The AIDS epidemic is not over. There is still a lot of work to do." - David Ho
- Historical Context: Late 20th century, the emergence of the HIV/AIDS pandemic, a time of fear, stigma, and urgent need for treatment.
- Early Life & Influences: Taiwanese-American physician and virologist, deeply involved in HIV/AIDS research from the early days of the epidemic.
- Major Contributions:
  - Pioneered the use of combination antiretroviral therapy (ART): This "cocktail" of drugs dramatically changed the course of HIV infection, turning it from a death sentence into a manageable chronic condition.
- Challenges & Controversies: Early HIV/AIDS drugs had significant side effects, the high cost of ART limited access in many parts of the world.
- Global Impact & Legacy:
  - His work has saved millions of lives and transformed the way HIV/AIDS is treated.
  - Continues to advocate for research on a cure and for better access to treatment globally.
- "Beyond the Scalpel": Ho has spoken out about the stigma faced by people living with HIV/AIDS, working to increase awareness and understanding.

## 36. Paul Farmer (USA): The Champion of Global Health Equity

- Opening Quote: "The idea that some lives matter less is the root of all that is wrong with the world." – Paul Farmer

- Historical Context: Late 20th and early 21st century, growing awareness of health disparities and the need for a global approach to health equity.
- Early Life & Influences: American physician and anthropologist, dedicated to providing healthcare to the poorest and most vulnerable populations.
- Major Contributions:
    - Co-founded Partners In Health (PIH): An organization that delivers healthcare in some of the poorest parts of the world, including Haiti, Rwanda, and Peru.
    - Advocate for social justice: Championed the idea that healthcare is a human right and worked to address the social determinants of health (poverty, lack of access to clean water, etc.).
- Challenges & Controversies: Criticized by some for focusing on resource-intensive care in poor settings, rather than more cost-effective public health measures.
- Global Impact & Legacy:
    - His work has inspired a generation of global health practitioners and advocates.
    - His writings on health equity and social justice have influenced policy and practice.
- "Beyond the Scalpel": Farmer lived a simple life, dedicating his time and resources to serving others.

### 37. Ben Carson (USA): Renowned Neurosurgeon
- Opening Quote: "Success is determined not by whether or not you face obstacles, but by your reaction to them. And if you look at these obstacles as a containing fence, they become your prison; but if you look at them as hurdles, each one strengthens you for the next." - Ben Carson
- Historical Context: Late 20th century, advancements in surgical techniques and imaging technology expanded the possibilities of neurosurgery.
- Early Life & Influences: Overcame a challenging childhood in Detroit to become a world-renowned pediatric neurosurgeon.
- Major Contributions:
    - Pioneered hemispherectomy: A radical procedure to remove half of the brain in children with severe epilepsy.
    - Led a team to successfully separate conjoined twins: A complex and risky procedure that highlighted his surgical skill.
- Challenges & Controversies: Later in life, his political views and public statements have generated controversy.
- Global Impact & Legacy:
    - His surgical innovations improved the lives of countless children with neurological disorders.
- "Beyond the Scalpel": Carson was known for his quiet demeanor, deep faith, and his belief in the power of hard work and education to overcome adversity.

## 38. Elizabeth Garrett Anderson (England): A Trailblazer for Women in Medicine
- Opening Quote: "Women must claim their right to take part in the administration of the world's work equally with men." – Elizabeth Garrett Anderson
- Historical Context: 19th-century England, strong opposition to women entering the medical profession.
- Early Life & Influences: Determined to become a doctor despite societal barriers, inspired by Elizabeth Blackwell's achievements in the USA.
- Major Contributions:
  - First woman to qualify as a physician and surgeon in Britain (1865).
  - Founded the New Hospital for Women in London: Staffed entirely by women, providing care and training for women.
- Challenges & Controversies: Faced constant opposition from the medical establishment, forced to find alternative routes to qualification.
- Global Impact & Legacy:
  - A pioneer for women's rights and medical education.
  - Her work opened doors for women to enter medicine and other professions.
- "Beyond the Scalpel": Garrett Anderson was also a prominent suffragist, campaigning for women's right to vote.

## 39. Wilhelm Conrad Röntgen (Germany): The Discoverer of X-rays
- Opening Quote: "I have not the slightest idea... but it is a kind of radiation." – Wilhelm Conrad Röntgen on his discovery of X-rays.
- Historical Context: Late 19th century, a time of great discoveries in physics, particularly in the study of electromagnetic radiation.
- Early Life & Influences: German physicist, experimenting with cathode rays, made a serendipitous discovery that would change medicine forever.
- Major Contributions:
  - Discovered X-rays in 1895: Found that a new type of radiation could penetrate solid objects, allowing visualization of the internal structures of the body.
- Challenges & Controversies: The dangers of radiation exposure were not fully understood until later.
- Global Impact & Legacy:
  - X-rays revolutionized medical diagnosis, enabling doctors to see broken bones, detect tumors, and diagnose a wide range of conditions.
  - His discovery continues to be essential in medical imaging today.
- "Beyond the Scalpel": Röntgen refused to patent his discovery, believing that knowledge should benefit all of humanity.

## 40. Sir William Osler (Canada): The Father of Modern Medicine

- Opening Quote: "The good physician treats the disease; the great physician treats the patient who has the disease." – William Osler
- Historical Context: Late 19th and early 20th centuries, a time of transition from traditional medicine to a more scientific approach.
- Early Life & Influences: Canadian physician, a brilliant clinician and teacher, emphasized bedside teaching and the importance of humanism in medicine.
- Major Contributions:
  - The Principles and Practice of Medicine (1892): A highly influential textbook that emphasized a scientific approach to diagnosis and treatment.
  - Promoted bedside teaching: Believed that medical students learned best by observing and interacting with patients.
- Challenges & Controversies: Some of his views on aging and euthanasia were considered controversial.
- Global Impact & Legacy:
  - Shaped medical education, emphasizing the importance of clinical skills, lifelong learning, and compassion.
  - His influence on medical humanism continues to be felt today.
- "Beyond the Scalpel": Osler was an avid collector of books and manuscripts, amassing a vast library on the history of medicine.

### 41. Karl Landsteiner (Austria): Discoverer of Blood Groups

- Opening Quote: "The blood of human beings is different." - Karl Landsteiner
- Historical Context: Early 20th century, blood transfusions were often fatal due to incompatible blood types.
- Early Life & Influences: Austrian biologist and physician, fascinated by the differences in human blood.
- Major Contributions:
  - Discovered the ABO blood groups in 1900: His work made safe blood transfusions possible.
- Challenges & Controversies: It took time for his discovery to be widely accepted and implemented.
- Global Impact & Legacy:
  - His work revolutionized blood transfusions, saving countless lives.
  - His research laid the foundation for understanding blood compatibility and transfusion medicine.
- "Beyond the Scalpel": Landsteiner also discovered the Rh factor in blood, another important factor in blood compatibility.

### 42. Harvey Cushing (USA): The Father of Neurosurgery

- Opening Quote: "The surgeon must have nerves of steel, the heart of a lion, and the hands of a lady." – Harvey Cushing
- Historical Context: Early 20th century, brain surgery was in its infancy, high mortality rates and limited techniques.
- Early Life & Influences: American neurosurgeon, a brilliant surgeon and meticulous researcher.
- Major Contributions:

- - o   Pioneered many neurosurgical techniques: Developed instruments and procedures for brain surgery, reducing mortality rates.
  - o   Detailed studies of brain tumors: Advanced the understanding and treatment of pituitary tumors and other brain lesions.
- Challenges & Controversies: His focus on surgical perfection sometimes came at the cost of patient relationships.
- Global Impact & Legacy:
  - o   Transformed neurosurgery from a risky and crude procedure into a more precise and effective specialty.
  - o   His work laid the foundation for modern neurosurgical practice.
- "Beyond the Scalpel": Cushing was an avid collector of medical books and artifacts, his collection formed the basis of the Harvey Cushing/John Hay Whitney Medical Library at Yale University.

### 43. Howard Florey (Australia) and Ernst Boris Chain (Germany): Developers of Penicillin Therapy

- Opening Quote: "Chance favors the prepared mind." – Louis Pasteur (a quote that applies to Florey and Chain's work building upon Fleming's discovery)
- Historical Context: World War II, a desperate need for treatments for bacterial infections.
- Early Life & Influences: Florey, an Australian pharmacologist; Chain, a German-born biochemist; they worked together at Oxford University to turn penicillin into a usable drug.
- Major Contributions:
  - o   Developed methods to purify and mass-produce penicillin: Turning Fleming's discovery into a life-saving treatment.
- Challenges & Controversies: The initial production of penicillin was difficult and time-consuming.
- Global Impact & Legacy:
  - o   Their work made penicillin widely available, saving millions of lives during the war and in the postwar era.
  - o   Credited with turning penicillin into a practical drug, paving the way for the antibiotic era.
- "Beyond the Scalpel": Both men were modest and dedicated scientists, driven by the desire to use their skills to improve human health.

### 44. Selman Waksman (Ukraine/USA): The Discoverer of Streptomycin

- Opening Quote: "The soil, it appears, is the greatest source of antibiotics." - Selman Waksman
- Historical Context: Mid-20th century, the search for new antibiotics to combat bacterial infections, particularly tuberculosis.
- Early Life & Influences: Ukrainian-American microbiologist and biochemist, dedicated to studying soil microorganisms.
- Major Contributions:

- - Discovered streptomycin in 1943: The first antibiotic effective against tuberculosis, a major breakthrough in the fight against this deadly disease.
  - Challenges & Controversies: There were legal disputes over patent rights for streptomycin.
  - Global Impact & Legacy:
    - Streptomycin saved millions of lives from tuberculosis and paved the way for the discovery of other antibiotics.
    - His work highlighted the importance of soil microbiology as a source of new drugs.
  - "Beyond the Scalpel": Waksman was a passionate teacher and mentor, inspiring generations of microbiologists.

### 45. Albert Sabin (Poland/USA): Developer of the Oral Polio Vaccine
- Opening Quote: "A scientist who is also a human being cannot rest while knowledge which might be used to reduce suffering is still unused." – Albert Sabin
- Historical Context: Mid-20th century, following the success of Salk's inactivated polio vaccine, the need for an even more effective vaccine to eradicate polio.
- Early Life & Influences: Polish-American medical researcher, dedicated to finding a way to stop polio.
- Major Contributions:
  - Developed the oral polio vaccine (OPV): Used a live, attenuated (weakened) virus, easier to administer and provided longer-lasting immunity.
- Challenges & Controversies: There were rare cases of vaccine-associated paralytic polio.
- Global Impact & Legacy:
  - The oral polio vaccine played a crucial role in the near-eradication of polio.
  - His work highlighted the importance of global vaccination campaigns.
- "Beyond the Scalpel": Sabin was a strong advocate for international cooperation in public health and believed that vaccines should be available to all children.

### 46. Gertrude B. Elion (USA): Pioneer in Drug Development
- Opening Quote: "Don't be afraid of hard work. Nothing worthwhile comes easily. Don't let others discourage you or tell you that you can't do it. In my day I was told women didn't go into chemistry. I saw no reason why we couldn't." – Gertrude B. Elion
- Historical Context: 20th century, the rise of pharmaceutical research and the development of new drugs to treat a wide range of diseases.
- Early Life & Influences: American biochemist and pharmacologist, faced discrimination as a woman in science, driven by the desire to develop new life-saving drugs.
- Major Contributions:
  - Developed numerous drugs: Including treatments for leukemia, malaria, gout, herpes, and organ transplant rejection.

- o Her work revolutionized drug development: Pioneered the use of rational drug design, tailoring drugs to specific biochemical targets.
- Challenges & Controversies: Some of the drugs she developed had side effects, the complex ethical considerations of drug development and testing.
- Global Impact & Legacy:
  - o Her discoveries have improved the lives of millions of people.
  - o Her work continues to inspire drug development today.
- "Beyond the Scalpel": Elion was a passionate advocate for science education, encouraging young people, especially women, to pursue careers in STEM fields.

## 47. Margaret Sanger (USA): A Controversial Champion: The Fight for Reproductive Rights and Access to Birth Control

- Opening Quote: "No woman can call herself free who does not own and control her body. No woman can call herself free until she can choose consciously whether she will or will not be a mother." - Margaret Sanger
- Historical Context: Early 20th century, a time when information about birth control was suppressed, and women had limited control over their reproductive health, leading to high rates of unwanted pregnancies and unsafe abortions.
- Early Life & Influences: American nurse and activist, witnessed firsthand the suffering caused by lack of access to birth control, particularly among poor women, dedicated her life to fighting for women's reproductive rights.
- Major Contributions:
  - o Founded the American Birth Control League (later Planned Parenthood): Provided information and access to contraception, empowering women to make informed choices about their reproductive health.
  - o Challenged Comstock Laws: Campaigned against laws that prohibited the distribution of information about birth control, facing arrest and legal challenges to advance her cause.
  - o Advocated for Women's Rights: Believed that access to birth control was essential for women's empowerment, social progress, and economic equality.
- Challenges & Controversies: Her work was met with strong opposition from religious groups, conservative politicians, and those who viewed birth control as immoral or a threat to traditional values. Her views on eugenics, though common in her time, are now widely condemned.
- Global Impact & Legacy: Her efforts transformed the landscape of reproductive health, paving the way for the legalization of birth control and increased access to family planning services.

- "Beyond the Scalpel": Sanger was a controversial figure, but her unwavering commitment to women's reproductive rights and her willingness to challenge societal norms have had a profound and lasting impact.

## 48. Hua Tuo (Ancient China): The Surgeon and Master of Anesthesia
- Opening Quote: "If the disease is located in the interior, it must be treated by an internal remedy." - Hua Tuo
- Historical Context: Han Dynasty China (206 BCE - 220 CE), Traditional Chinese Medicine (TCM) developing, with advancements in acupuncture, herbal remedies, and surgery.
- Early Life & Influences: A renowned physician and surgeon, traveled widely, known for his diagnostic skills and innovative treatments.
- Major Contributions:
    - Credited with developing "mafeisan" (possibly a form of surgical anesthesia): Allowed for painless surgery, a significant advancement.
    - Advocated for physical exercise and "wuqinxi" (five animal exercises): A form of therapeutic exercise, promoting health and well-being.
- Challenges & Controversies: Little concrete evidence exists about his anesthesia methods, his story is intertwined with legend.
- Global Impact & Legacy:
    - His contributions to surgery and anesthesia demonstrate the advancements of Chinese medicine in the ancient world.
    - His emphasis on exercise and movement influenced the development of martial arts and other forms of exercise in China.
- "Beyond the Scalpel": Hua Tuo's story reflects the importance of compassion and ethical conduct in medicine, as he is said to have treated both the rich and poor with equal care

## 49. Michael DeBakey (USA): The Master of Cardiovascular Surgery
- Opening Quote: "A heart surgeon should be a thinking man." - Michael DeBakey
- Historical Context: 20th century, advancements in surgery made complex cardiovascular procedures possible.
- Early Life & Influences: American surgeon, a pioneer in the development of open-heart surgery and vascular surgery.
- Major Contributions:
    - Developed techniques for repairing aortic aneurysms: Developed the roller pump, a key component of the heart-lung machine.
    - Performed some of the first coronary artery bypass surgeries: Extending the lives of patients with heart disease.

- Challenges & Controversies: Some of his early procedures were high-risk, faced ethical challenges as a medical innovator.
- Global Impact & Legacy:
  - His innovations transformed cardiovascular surgery and saved countless lives.
  - His influence on surgical training and research was profound.
- "Beyond the Scalpel": DeBakey was known for his long hours, rigorous work ethic, and commitment to improving patient care.

### 50. C. Walton Lillehei (USA): The Father of Open-Heart Surgery
- Opening Quote: "I had a sense that a great opportunity was being presented to me... to be involved in the very beginnings of an entirely new field of surgery that would benefit a great many people." – C. Walton Lillehei
- Historical Context: Mid-20th century, the challenge of operating on a beating heart was a major obstacle to cardiac surgery.
- Early Life & Influences: American surgeon, a pioneer in the development of open-heart surgery, a gifted innovator who solved complex problems.
- Major Contributions:
  - Developed the cross-circulation technique: Using a human donor (often a parent) as a temporary heart-lung machine, allowing for operations on the recipient's heart.
  - Pioneered the use of mechanical heart-lung machines: This made open-heart surgery more widely available.
- Challenges & Controversies: The cross-circulation technique was risky for both the patient and the donor, early heart-lung machines had limitations.
- Global Impact & Legacy:
  - His innovations made open-heart surgery possible, leading to the treatment of congenital heart defects and other cardiac conditions.
  - His work paved the way for the advancements in cardiac surgery that we see today.
- "Beyond the Scalpel": Lillehei was known for his supportive and collaborative approach, working closely with engineers and other specialists to solve problems.

### 51. Harold Gillies (New Zealand/England): The Father of Plastic Surgery
- Opening Quote: "Surgery is not carpentry, there is a soul there." – Harold Gillies
- Historical Context: World War I, devastating facial injuries from trench warfare created a need for innovative reconstructive surgery.
- Early Life & Influences: New Zealand-born surgeon who worked in England, dedicated to helping soldiers disfigured by war.
- Major Contributions:

- Developed many techniques in plastic surgery: Skin grafting, flap surgery, and reconstructive techniques for the face and jaw.
- Founded the Queen's Hospital, Sidcup: The first hospital dedicated to plastic surgery, a center of innovation.
- Challenges & Controversies: The psychological impact of disfigurement, the limits of reconstruction surgery in a time before microsurgery.
- Global Impact & Legacy:
  - Transformed the field of plastic surgery, his techniques have been refined and are still used today.
  - His work brought hope and restored dignity to countless patients.
- "Beyond the Scalpel": Gillies was known for his optimistic spirit and his belief in the ability of surgery to restore not only physical form but also self-esteem.

## 52. Willem Johan Kolff (Netherlands/USA): Pioneer of Artificial Organs

- Opening Quote: "Why should we not try to keep a man alive after his kidneys have failed?" - Willem Kolff
- Historical Context: Mid-20th century, the concept of replacing failing organs with artificial devices was a radical idea.
- Early Life & Influences: Dutch physician, witnessed the suffering of patients with kidney failure, determined to find a way to save their lives.
- Major Contributions:
  - Developed the first artificial kidney (hemodialysis machine) in 1943: His invention made long-term treatment of kidney failure possible.
  - Pioneered research on artificial hearts and other organs: Laid the foundation for the development of artificial organs.
- Challenges & Controversies: Early dialysis machines were bulky and inefficient, the ethical implications of artificial organ transplantation.
- Global Impact & Legacy:
  - His work revolutionized the treatment of kidney failure, allowing millions of people to live longer and healthier lives.
  - His innovations inspired further research in bioengineering and artificial organ development.
- "Beyond the Scalpel": Kolff was a visionary inventor, constantly seeking ways to improve the lives of patients facing life-threatening conditions.

## 53. Charles Richard Drew (USA): Pioneer of Blood Banking

- Opening Quote: "There is no such thing as 'black' blood or 'white' blood." – Charles Drew
- Historical Context: World War II, an urgent need for blood transfusions for wounded soldiers.

- Early Life & Influences: African American physician and surgeon, faced racial discrimination throughout his career, dedicated to improving access to healthcare.
- Major Contributions:
  - Developed methods for blood storage and preservation: His work led to the establishment of blood banks.
  - Organized blood drives: Collected and distributed blood for transfusions during the war.
- Challenges & Controversies: Challenged the racist policies of the American Red Cross, which initially segregated blood by race, his early death in a car accident is considered a tragic loss to medicine.
- Global Impact & Legacy:
  - His work revolutionized blood banking and transfusion medicine, saving countless lives.
  - His legacy continues to inspire efforts to improve blood safety and access to blood transfusions worldwide.
- "Beyond the Scalpel": Drew was a gifted athlete, a star football player in college, demonstrating his diverse talents.

## 54. Alfred Blalock (USA) and Vivien Thomas (USA): Pioneers of Cardiac Surgery

- Opening Quote: "Let's go in there and see what's going on." – Alfred Blalock, known for his bold surgical approach.
- Historical Context: Mid-20th century, limited understanding and treatment for congenital heart defects.
- Early Life & Influences: Blalock, a surgeon; Thomas, an African American surgical technician with extraordinary skills, but denied formal recognition due to racial discrimination.
- Major Contributions:
  - Developed the Blalock-Taussig shunt: A groundbreaking surgical procedure to improve blood flow to the lungs in children with "blue baby syndrome."
  - Their collaboration: A remarkable story of surgical innovation and the overcoming of racial barriers.
- Challenges & Controversies: Thomas' contributions were not fully acknowledged until much later, highlighting the injustices of racial segregation in medicine.
- Global Impact & Legacy:
  - The Blalock-Taussig shunt saved the lives of countless children with congenital heart defects.
  - Their work transformed pediatric cardiac surgery and set the stage for modern cardiac interventions.
- "Beyond the Scalpel": The story of Blalock and Thomas highlights the importance of collaboration, mentorship, and recognizing the contributions of all members of a surgical team.

## 55. Jonas Edward Salk (USA): The Visionary Researcher

- Opening Quote: "There is no patent. Could you patent the sun?" – Jonas Salk, on refusing to patent the polio vaccine.

- Historical Context: Following the success of the polio vaccine, the need to address other major health challenges and the ethical implications of scientific research.
- Early Life & Influences: American virologist, the developer of the polio vaccine, a thoughtful and philosophical scientist.
- Major Contributions:
  - Founded the Salk Institute for Biological Studies: A research center dedicated to exploring fundamental questions in biology and the human condition.
  - Wrote on biophilosophy: Explored the ethical and social implications of scientific advancements.
- Challenges & Controversies: His views on bioethics and population control were sometimes controversial.
- Global Impact & Legacy:
  - His work on polio inspired other vaccine development efforts.
  - His philosophical writings prompted reflection on the role of science in society.
- "Beyond the Scalpel": Salk was a Renaissance man with interests in art, music, and architecture, demonstrating a broad intellectual curiosity.

**56. Godfrey Hounsfield (England): The Architect of the CT Scan: Revolutionizing Medical Imaging**
- Opening Quote: "It wasn't a sudden inspiration... it was a gradual realization." - Godfrey Hounsfield, on the development of the CT scan.
- Historical Context: Mid-20th century, medical imaging was limited to X-rays, providing a two-dimensional view of the body's internal structures, the need for more detailed and three-dimensional imaging.
- Early Life & Influences: British electrical engineer, worked at EMI (Electric and Musical Industries), his interest in computer technology and pattern recognition led him to revolutionize medical imaging.
- Major Contributions:
  - Developed the first computed tomography (CT) scanner: His invention created detailed cross-sectional images of the body, providing a revolutionary new way to diagnose and monitor diseases.
- Challenges & Controversies: Early CT scanners were expensive and time-consuming, raising concerns about access and cost-effectiveness. The use of ionizing radiation in CT scans raised questions about potential risks.
- Global Impact & Legacy: The CT scan has transformed medical diagnostics, becoming an essential tool in the diagnosis and management of a wide range of conditions, from strokes and tumors to fractures and infections.
- "Beyond the Scalpel": Hounsfield was a self-taught engineer with a passion for solving complex problems, demonstrating the power of interdisciplinary thinking and innovation in medicine.

## 57. Aubrey Levin (South Africa/Canada): A Controversial Legacy
- Opening Quote: [Omit a quote due to the controversial nature of this figure. The chapter will need to acknowledge the complexities of Levin's legacy directly.]
- Historical Context: 20th century, the abuse of power by medical professionals and the use of unethical practices.
- Early Life & Influences: South African-born Canadian psychiatrist, specializing in sexual dysfunction, held positions of authority, but his practices would later come under scrutiny.
- Major Contributions:
  - [Focus on his early, legitimate work in psychiatry if possible.]
  - [The chapter must address his later conviction for sexual assault of patients, this is unavoidable.]
- Challenges & Controversies: His career ended in disgrace due to his criminal conviction, raising questions about the abuse of power in healthcare settings and the need for accountability.
- Global Impact & Legacy:
  - His case serves as a cautionary tale, highlighting the importance of medical ethics and the need to protect vulnerable patients.
- "Beyond the Scalpel": The inclusion of this chapter is intended to provoke discussion and reflection on the darker side of medicine and the abuse of trust.

## 58. William DeVries (USA): The Artificial Heart Innovator
- Opening Quote: "The purpose of the artificial heart is not to make man immortal, but to make living with a failing heart more bearable." - William DeVries
- Historical Context: Late 20th century, the quest to develop artificial organs to replace failing hearts.
- Early Life & Influences: American surgeon, a pioneer in the field of artificial hearts, trained under Willem Kolff (the developer of the artificial kidney).
- Major Contributions:
  - Implanted the first permanent artificial heart (Jarvik-7) in 1982: The patient, Barney Clark, lived for 112 days, a significant milestone in artificial organ development.
- Challenges & Controversies: Early artificial hearts had limitations and complications, ethical concerns about the use of artificial organs to prolong life.
- Global Impact & Legacy:
  - His work advanced the development of artificial hearts, which are now used as temporary life support or as a bridge to transplantation.
  - His work sparked debate about the ethical implications of extending life through technology.

- "Beyond the Scalpel": DeVries faced immense pressure and scrutiny during the first artificial heart implant, his courage and determination were tested during that time.

## 59. Robert Gallo (USA): The Co-Discoverer of HIV
- Opening Quote: "The discovery of HIV was a major milestone in our understanding of AIDS, but it was only the beginning of a long and difficult journey." – Robert Gallo
- Historical Context: Early 1980s, the identification of the virus that causes AIDS, a major breakthrough in the fight against the pandemic.
- Early Life & Influences: American biomedical researcher, dedicated to studying retroviruses, his laboratory was key to isolating and identifying HIV.
- Major Contributions:
    - Independently discovered the human immunodeficiency virus (HIV) in 1984: His work led to the development of blood tests to screen for HIV.
- Challenges & Controversies: Dispute with Luc Montagnier's team in France over who first discovered the virus, the patent dispute over the HIV blood test.
- Global Impact & Legacy:
    - His work was essential in understanding the cause of AIDS, leading to the development of treatments and prevention strategies.
- "Beyond the Scalpel": Gallo faced criticism for his handling of the patent dispute, but his contributions to HIV/AIDS research are undeniable.

## 60. Luc Montagnier (France): Co-Discoverer of HIV
- Opening Quote: "It's not my fault if the Americans were slow. They're too obsessed with their Nobel Prize." - Luc Montagnier, commenting on the controversy over the discovery of HIV.
- Historical Context: The early 1980s, the global HIV/AIDS epidemic was emerging, the race to identify the cause of the disease.
- Early Life & Influences: French virologist, director of the Pasteur Institute in Paris, his research team was the first to isolate and identify the virus that causes AIDS.
- Major Contributions:
    - His research team was the first to identify the human immunodeficiency virus (HIV) in 1983: Their discovery paved the way for the development of blood tests and treatments.
- Challenges & Controversies: Dispute with Robert Gallo's team over the credit for the discovery of HIV.
- Global Impact & Legacy:
    - His work was critical in understanding the origins and mechanisms of HIV infection, leading to the development of life-saving treatments.
- "Beyond the Scalpel": Montagnier's later research on electromagnetic signals from DNA generated controversy and skepticism within the scientific community.

## 61. Anthony Fauci (USA): The Face of Infectious Disease Research
- Opening Quote: "You always have to stay ahead of the curve in infectious diseases." – Anthony Fauci
- Historical Context: Late 20th and early 21st century, emerging infectious diseases like HIV/AIDS, Ebola, and COVID-19 pose major threats to global health.
- Early Life & Influences: American physician and immunologist, a leading expert on infectious diseases, director of the National Institute of Allergy and Infectious Diseases (NIAID) since 1984.
- Major Contributions:
    - Led research on HIV/AIDS: His work was critical in understanding the disease and developing effective treatments.
    - Advised multiple presidents on infectious disease outbreaks: A key figure in the response to HIV/AIDS, Ebola, Zika, and COVID-19.
- Challenges & Controversies: Navigating the political complexities of public health, facing criticism during the COVID-19 pandemic.
- Global Impact & Legacy:
    - His leadership has shaped the U.S. response to infectious diseases and influenced global health policy.
    - His calm and science-based approach has made him a trusted voice during public health crises.
- "Beyond the Scalpel": Fauci is known for his dedication to science, his long work hours, and his commitment to mentoring young scientists.

## 62. Jane Cooke Wright (USA): A Pioneer in Cancer Chemotherapy
- Opening Quote: "There is no greater joy, nor greater reward than to make a fundamental difference in someone's life." - Jane Cooke Wright
- Historical Context: Mid-20th century, cancer treatment was in its early stages, chemotherapy was a developing field.
- Early Life & Influences: African American physician and researcher, daughter of a prominent surgeon, dedicated to improving cancer treatment, particularly for underserved populations.
- Major Contributions:
    - Pioneered research in chemotherapy: Developed new chemotherapy drugs and methods for delivering them more effectively.
    - Studied the use of methotrexate: A drug that became widely used in cancer treatment.
- Challenges & Controversies: Faced racial and gender discrimination in medicine, struggled to secure funding for her research.
- Global Impact & Legacy:
    - Her work advanced the field of chemotherapy and improved outcomes for cancer patients.
    - She was a role model for African American women in science and medicine.

- "Beyond the Scalpel": Wright was known for her compassion for her patients and her belief in the importance of equal access to healthcare.

## 63. Harold Varmus (USA): Decoding the Genetic Origins of Cancer
### Harold Varmus (USA): From the Lab to the NIH
- Opening Quote: "The pursuit of knowledge is a noble and worthy endeavor." - Harold Varmus
- Historical Context: Late 20th century, advances in molecular biology and genetics, a growing understanding of the genetic basis of diseases, including cancer.
- Early Life & Influences: American scientist and Nobel laureate, his research on oncogenes transformed our understanding of cancer.
- Major Contributions:
    - Served as Director of the National Institutes of Health (NIH) from 1993 to 1999: Oversaw a period of significant growth in medical research and funding.
    - Advocated for open access to scientific publications: Believed that scientific knowledge should be shared widely to accelerate progress.
- Challenges & Controversies: Balancing the demands of scientific research with the complexities of government bureaucracy, ethical issues surrounding gene therapy and genetic testing.
- Global Impact & Legacy:
    - His leadership at the NIH helped to advance medical research and improve health outcomes.
    - His advocacy for open access to scientific information has facilitated scientific collaboration and progress.
- "Beyond the Scalpel": Varmus is a passionate advocate for science education and literacy, believing that a greater understanding of science is essential for an informed citizenry.

## 64. Elizabeth Kenny (Australia): Challenging Conventional Polio Treatment
- Opening Quote: "He can walk because I would not let him lie still." - Elizabeth Kenny, on her innovative approach to polio treatment.
- Historical Context: Early 20th century, polio epidemics were causing widespread fear and paralysis, conventional treatment often involved immobilization, which could worsen outcomes.
- Early Life & Influences: Australian nurse, developed her own methods for treating polio based on observation and intuition, challenged medical dogma.
- Major Contributions:
    - Developed the "Kenny Method": Focused on muscle re-education, hot packs, and exercise, rather than immobilization, her methods proved more effective in restoring function.
- Challenges & Controversies: Faced strong resistance from the medical establishment, her methods were initially dismissed and ridiculed.

- Global Impact & Legacy:
  - Her innovative approach to polio treatment transformed the field, her methods were eventually adopted and are still used in physical therapy today.
  - Her work highlighted the importance of challenging conventional wisdom and the value of a patient-centered approach.
- "Beyond the Scalpel": Kenny was a strong-willed and independent woman who fought tirelessly to gain acceptance for her methods, eventually gaining international recognition for her work.

## 65 Harold Freeman (USA): A Lifetime of Service: Building a Model for Cancer Care Equity

- **Opening Quote:** "Healthcare is a right, not a privilege." - Harold Freeman
- **Historical Context:** Late 20th and early 21st century, increasing awareness of racial disparities in cancer care and outcomes, the need for community-based solutions to address healthcare inequities.
- **Early Life & Influences:** African American surgeon and oncologist, a leading advocate for eliminating disparities in cancer care, dedicated to serving underserved communities and improving access to cancer screening and treatment.
- **Major Contributions:**
- **Founded the Ralph Lauren Center for Cancer Care and Prevention in Harlem:** A model for providing culturally sensitive, high-quality cancer care in an underserved community, integrating medical treatment with social support services.
- **Developed the "Patient Navigation" Model:** Recognizing the complexities of the healthcare system, he created a model that uses trained navigators to guide patients through the process of diagnosis, treatment, and follow-up care, helping to overcome barriers to access.
- **Challenges & Controversies:** Addressing the systemic and persistent nature of racial disparities in healthcare, securing funding for programs to support underserved communities, and advocating for policy changes to promote health equity.
- **Global Impact & Legacy:** His work has helped to reduce disparities in cancer care and improve outcomes for minority patients. His legacy continues to inspire efforts to achieve health equity for all and to develop innovative models of care delivery in underserved communities.
- **"Beyond the Scalpel":** Freeman was a compassionate and tireless advocate for his patients, working to empower them and ensure their access to quality healthcare throughout his career.

## 66. Helen Taussig (USA): A Lifetime of Advocacy for Children with Heart Defects

- Opening Quote: "The more I learned, the more I saw how little I knew, how much more there was to learn." - Helen Taussig

- Historical Context: Mid-20th century, growing understanding of congenital heart defects and the development of surgical treatments.
- Early Life & Influences: American cardiologist, dedicated to helping children with heart defects, her own hearing loss instilled empathy for patients facing challenges.
- Major Contributions:
  - Founded the field of pediatric cardiology: Her research and clinical work focused on the diagnosis and treatment of heart defects in children.
  - Established clinics and programs: Devoted her life to improving the care and lives of children with heart disease.
- Challenges & Controversies: Gender discrimination in the medical field, ethical considerations of performing complex surgeries on young children.
- Global Impact & Legacy:
  - Her work saved countless lives and transformed the way children with heart defects are treated.
  - Her legacy continues to inspire pediatric cardiologists and advocates for children with disabilities.
- "Beyond the Scalpel": Taussig was a gifted teacher and mentor, inspiring generations of medical students and cardiologists, known for her patience and generosity.

## 67. Al-Zahrawi (Abulcasis) (Islamic Spain): The Father of Modern Surgery in Europe

- Opening Quote: "Surgery is the last resort." – Al-Zahrawi
- Historical Context: Islamic Golden Age in Spain (10th-11th centuries), a time of flourishing intellectual and scientific activity, particularly in medicine.
- Early Life & Influences: Born in Cordoba, Spain, served as a court physician, renowned surgeon, his work bridged the knowledge of the East and West.
- Major Contributions:
  - Al-Tasrif (The Method of Medicine): A 30-volume medical encyclopedia, including a detailed treatise on surgery (Kitab al-Tasrif), introduced surgical instruments and techniques to Europe.
- Challenges & Controversies: His work challenged the prevailing medical practices in Europe, which were lagging behind those in the Islamic world.
- Global Impact & Legacy:
  - Al-Tasrif was translated into Latin and became a standard surgical text in Europe for centuries.
  - His work laid the foundation for the development of modern surgery in Europe, bridging the gap between ancient and Renaissance medicine.
- "Beyond the Scalpel": Al-Zahrawi emphasized the importance of ethics in surgery, advocating for compassion, gentleness, and careful observation.

## 68. Jean-Martin Charcot (France): The Architect of Modern Neurology
- Opening Quote: "The greatest danger for most of us is not that our aim is too high and we miss it, but that it is too low and we reach it." - Jean-Martin Charcot
- Historical Context: Late 19th century, neurology was emerging as a distinct medical specialty, limited understanding of neurological disorders, a need for systematic classification and treatment.
- Early Life & Influences: French neurologist, his work at the Salpêtrière Hospital in Paris transformed the understanding and treatment of neurological disorders.
- Major Contributions:
- Systematic study of neurological diseases: His detailed descriptions and classifications of conditions like multiple sclerosis, amyotrophic lateral sclerosis (ALS), and Parkinson's disease laid the foundation for modern neurology.
- Pioneer in the study of hysteria: His work on hysteria, while controversial, contributed to the understanding of psychological disorders and the mind-body connection.
- Challenges & Controversies: His public demonstrations of hypnosis on female patients with hysteria were criticized as exploitative and theatrical, raising questions about medical ethics and the treatment of vulnerable patients.
- Global Impact & Legacy:
- His contributions to neurology were profound, his descriptions of diseases and his classifications are still used today.
- His work influenced Sigmund Freud and other early pioneers in psychiatry and psychology.
- "Beyond the Scalpel": Charcot was a gifted artist and a passionate collector of anatomical specimens and medical artifacts, reflecting his interest in the beauty and complexity of the human body.
-

## 69. C. Walton Lillehei (USA): The Mentor and the Legacy Builder
- Opening Quote: "The most important thing in medicine is to teach the next generation." - C. Walton Lillehei
- Historical Context: Following the development of open-heart surgery, the need for training and education to spread these life-saving techniques.
- Early Life & Influences: American cardiac surgeon, pioneer of open-heart surgery, known for his surgical skill and his dedication to teaching.
- Major Contributions:
  - Trained generations of cardiac surgeons: His trainees went on to establish prominent cardiac surgery programs around the world.
  - Founded the Lillehei Heart Institute: A center for research and innovation in cardiovascular care.

- Challenges & Controversies: The high risks and technical challenges of early open-heart surgery, ethical considerations of experimental surgical techniques.
- Global Impact & Legacy:
    - His legacy extends far beyond his own surgical innovations, his students carried his techniques and philosophy to other parts of the world.
    - His mentorship model emphasized collaboration, creativity, and a commitment to patient care.
- "Beyond the Scalpel": Lillehei was known for his humble personality and his commitment to teamwork, recognizing the contributions of all members of the surgical team.

## 70. Harold Gillies (New Zealand/England): A Legacy of Restoring Lives

- Opening Quote: "A plastic surgeon is an artist, but his materials are living flesh and blood." - Harold Gillies
- Historical Context: Following World War I, the growing need for reconstructive surgery to treat war injuries and other disfiguring conditions.
- Early Life & Influences: New Zealand-born surgeon who worked in England, pioneer in the field of plastic surgery, dedicated to restoring the lives of those with facial injuries.
- Major Contributions:
    - Established the field of plastic surgery: His innovative techniques and dedication to reconstructive surgery shaped the specialty.
    - Founded the British Association of Plastic Surgeons: Promoted the advancement and recognition of plastic surgery.
- Challenges & Controversies: The psychological impact of facial disfigurement on soldiers and civilians, the limitations of surgical techniques before the advent of microsurgery.
- Global Impact & Legacy:
    - His work has inspired generations of plastic surgeons and improved the lives of countless patients.
    - His contributions to reconstructive surgery have applications in treating burns, trauma, and congenital deformities.
- "Beyond the Scalpel": Gillies was known for his warm and compassionate personality, his ability to connect with his patients and understand their needs.

## 71. Willem Johan Kolff (Netherlands/USA): The Artificial Organ Visionary

- Opening Quote: "I have a strong feeling that artificial organs are here to stay and that they will multiply and increase in importance." – Willem Kolff
- Historical Context: 20th century, the development of bioengineering and the quest to develop artificial organs to replace failing body systems.

- Early Life & Influences: Dutch physician and inventor, driven by the desire to find ways to support failing organs and save lives.
- Major Contributions:
  - Continued to innovate artificial organs: Developed the first artificial heart in 1957, a prototype for future designs.
  - Founded the American Society for Artificial Internal Organs (ASAIO): Promoting research and development of artificial organs.
- Challenges & Controversies: Early artificial organs had limitations and complications, the high costs and ethical considerations of artificial organ transplantation.
- Global Impact & Legacy:
  - His visionary work inspired generations of bioengineers and medical researchers.
  - His innovations have led to the development of life-saving artificial organs, including hearts, lungs, and kidneys.
- "Beyond the Scalpel": Kolff was a tireless advocate for artificial organ research and believed that technology could be used to extend and improve human life.

## 72. Charles Richard Drew (USA): A Legacy of Blood and Equality

- Opening Quote: [Use a quote that highlights Drew's advocacy for racial equality in healthcare.]
- Historical Context: Mid-20th century, racial segregation in the United States, limited access to healthcare for African Americans.
- Early Life & Influences: African American surgeon, pioneer in blood banking, faced discrimination, determined to use his skills to serve all people.
- Major Contributions:
  - Directed the blood plasma program for the American Red Cross during World War II: Ensuring the availability of blood for transfusions, saving countless lives.
  - Challenged racial segregation in blood donation: Argued that there was no scientific basis for separating blood by race.
- Challenges & Controversies: His resignation from the Red Cross in protest of their discriminatory blood donation policies.
- Global Impact & Legacy:
  - His work helped to dismantle racist policies in blood banking and make blood transfusions safer.
  - His legacy continues to inspire efforts to achieve health equity and eliminate racial disparities in healthcare.
- "Beyond the Scalpel": Drew was a gifted athlete and a scholar, demonstrating his diverse talents and his commitment to excellence.

## 73. Alfred Blalock (USA): The Southern Surgeon Who Challenged Norms

- Opening Quote: "Don't be afraid to take risks. Sometimes the biggest rewards come from taking the biggest chances." - Alfred Blalock
- Historical Context: Mid-20th century, racial segregation in the U.S. South, limited opportunities for African Americans in medicine.
- Early Life & Influences: American surgeon, known for his boldness in the operating room, challenged racial barriers by working with Vivien Thomas, an African American surgical technician.
- Major Contributions:
    - Continued to innovate in cardiac surgery: Developed new techniques for treating shock and other surgical conditions.
    - Mentored Vivien Thomas: Gave Thomas opportunities to develop his surgical skills, a testament to his willingness to defy racial norms.
- Challenges & Controversies: The limited recognition given to Vivien Thomas during their time, the ethical complexities of experimental surgery.
- Global Impact & Legacy:
    - His work advanced cardiac surgery and paved the way for future innovations.
    - His partnership with Thomas was a step toward greater inclusivity in medicine, but it also highlighted the persistent injustices of racial discrimination.
- "Beyond the Scalpel": Blalock was known for his strong personality, demanding standards, and his dedication to advancing surgical techniques.

## 74. Selman Waksman (Ukraine/USA): The Soil and the Search for Antibiotics

- Opening Quote: "Antibiotics... have given man the power to conquer many of the dread diseases that have plagued him since the dawn of history." - Selman Waksman
- Historical Context: Following the discovery of penicillin and streptomycin, the need for new antibiotics to combat bacterial infections and drug resistance.
- Early Life & Influences: Ukrainian-American microbiologist and biochemist, dedicated to exploring the world of soil microorganisms as a source of new drugs.
- Major Contributions:
    - Discovered several other antibiotics: Including neomycin, which is still used today in topical medications.
    - Developed methods for screening soil microbes for antibiotic activity: His work laid the foundation for the modern pharmaceutical industry's search for new drugs.
- Challenges & Controversies: The emergence of antibiotic resistance, the ecological impact of antibiotic use, the complex ethical considerations of drug development.
- Global Impact & Legacy:
    - His work has led to the discovery of numerous antibiotics that have saved countless lives.

- o His legacy continues to inspire research into new antimicrobial agents.
- "Beyond the Scalpel": Waksman was a passionate advocate for the conservation of soil resources and the importance of protecting the natural world.

## 75. Albert Sabin (Poland/USA): Eradicating Polio, a Global Effort
- Opening Quote: "My only regret is that we did not succeed in eradicating polio in my lifetime." – Albert Sabin
- Historical Context: Following the introduction of the oral polio vaccine, the worldwide effort to eradicate polio, the challenges of global vaccination campaigns.
- Early Life & Influences: Polish-American medical researcher, dedicated to controlling infectious diseases, a tireless advocate for global health.
- Major Contributions:
  - o Led the effort to eradicate polio: His oral polio vaccine played a crucial role in reducing the incidence of polio worldwide.
  - o Worked with the World Health Organization (WHO): To implement mass vaccination campaigns, particularly in developing countries.
- Challenges & Controversies: Obstacles to polio eradication in conflict zones and regions with limited healthcare access, concerns about vaccine safety.
- Global Impact & Legacy:
  - o His work has brought the world closer to eradicating polio, saving millions of children from paralysis and death.
  - o His legacy continues to inspire global health efforts to eliminate infectious diseases.
- "Beyond the Scalpel": Sabin was a humanist who believed that science should be used to serve humanity, particularly the most vulnerable.

## 76. Gertrude B. Elion (USA): The Power of Rational Drug Design
- Opening Quote: "The more basic research that is done, the more possibilities for applications." – Gertrude B. Elion
- Historical Context: 20th century, the rapid growth of pharmaceutical research, the development of more targeted and effective drugs.
- Early Life & Influences: American biochemist and pharmacologist, a pioneer in the field of rational drug design, driven by a passion to improve the lives of patients.
- Major Contributions:
  - o Continued to develop innovative drugs: Her work led to treatments for immune disorders, viral infections, and organ transplant rejection.
  - o Advanced the field of rational drug design: Her approach focused on understanding the specific biochemical pathways involved in disease, allowing for the creation of drugs tailored to specific targets.

- Challenges & Controversies: The high cost of developing new drugs, the ethical considerations of drug testing and access.
- Global Impact & Legacy:
  - Her work has revolutionized drug development, leading to more effective and safer medications.
  - Her discoveries have improved the lives of millions of people with various diseases.
- "Beyond the Scalpel": Elion was a dedicated mentor to young scientists and a strong advocate for women in science.

### 77. Denton Cooley (USA): A Giant of Cardiac Surgery
- Opening Quote: "The heart is a muscle like any other; it can be trained and strengthened." – Denton Cooley
- Historical Context: 20th century, the rapid development of cardiac surgery, pushing the boundaries of what was surgically possible.
- Early Life & Influences: American cardiac surgeon, known for his innovative techniques and his boldness in the operating room, a pioneer in heart transplantation.
- Major Contributions:
  - Performed the first successful implantation of a total artificial heart in the US (1969): Used as a bridge to transplantation, a major step in artificial organ development.
  - Developed techniques for repairing aortic aneurysms: Advanced the field of vascular surgery.
- Challenges & Controversies: Ethical questions surrounding the use of artificial hearts, the allocation of scarce donor organs, his competitive rivalry with Michael DeBakey.
- Global Impact & Legacy:
  - His work has saved the lives of countless patients with heart disease.
  - His influence on cardiac surgery continues to be felt today.
- "Beyond the Scalpel": Cooley was a skilled pianist and a pilot, showcasing his diverse talents and his passion for pushing boundaries.

### 78. Imhotep (Ancient Egypt): The God-Physician
- Opening Quote: "I have heard the words of Imhotep and Hardedef, with whose sayings men speak so much." – From the Papyrus Prisse, an ancient Egyptian text.
- Historical Context: Old Kingdom Egypt (c. 2686–2181 BCE), medicine intertwined with religion and magic. Imhotep served as vizier to Pharaoh Djoser and was renowned for his wisdom in medicine, architecture, and engineering.
- Early Life & Influences: Little is known with certainty, but his legend grew over time. He was deified after his death, revered as a god of healing and wisdom.
- Major Contributions:
  - Attributed with the Edwin Smith Papyrus: A surgical treatise containing rational and practical treatments for wounds and injuries.

- Credited with designing the Step Pyramid of Djoser: Showcasing his knowledge of architecture and engineering.
- Challenges & Controversies: Separating fact from legend is challenging, as his life became intertwined with mythology.
- Global Impact & Legacy:
  - Represented the advancement of medicine in ancient Egypt, a civilization that made significant contributions to surgery, anatomy, and pharmacology.
  - His influence on Egyptian culture and religion highlights the interconnectedness of medicine and spirituality.
- "Beyond the Scalpel": Imhotep was a polymath, a master of multiple disciplines, symbolizing the pursuit of knowledge in ancient Egypt.

### 79. Thomas Starzl (USA): The Father of Modern Transplantation

- Opening Quote: "Transplantation is not just a science; it's an art, a philosophy, and a humanitarian endeavor." - Thomas Starzl
- Historical Context: 20th century, the development of immunosuppressive drugs made organ transplantation more successful, the need to overcome organ rejection.
- Early Life & Influences: American surgeon, a pioneer in liver transplantation, dedicated to improving transplant techniques and outcomes.
- Major Contributions:
  - Performed the first successful human liver transplant: In 1963, his work paved the way for liver transplantation to become a standard treatment.
  - Developed immunosuppressive regimens: Reduced the risk of organ rejection, a key to successful transplantation.
- Challenges & Controversies: Early transplant surgeries were high-risk, ethical concerns about organ allocation and the cost of transplant surgery.
- Global Impact & Legacy:
  - Transformed the field of organ transplantation, his work led to the development of transplant centers around the world.
  - His legacy continues to inspire research in transplant immunology and organ preservation.
- "Beyond the Scalpel": Starzl was known for his tireless work ethic, his unwavering commitment to his patients, and his belief in the transformative power of transplantation.

### 80. Patch Adams (USA): The Doctor of Laughter

- Opening Quote: "We've got to start treating people as human beings, not as a diagnosis." - Patch Adams
- Historical Context: Late 20th century, growing awareness of the importance of holistic care and the role of humor and compassion in healing.

- Early Life & Influences: American physician and social activist, a strong advocate for humanism in medicine, believed in the power of laughter to promote health and well-being.
- Major Contributions:
  - Founded the Gesundheit! Institute: A free community hospital based on the principles of holistic care, humor, and compassion.
  - Promoted the therapeutic value of laughter: His clown doctor approach brought joy and laughter to hospitalized children and adults.
- Challenges & Controversies: His unconventional methods and philosophy have been criticized by some in the traditional medical community.
- Global Impact & Legacy:
  - His work has inspired others to incorporate humor and play into healthcare settings.
  - His legacy continues to advocate for a more human and compassionate approach to medicine.
- "Beyond the Scalpel": Adams is known for his colorful personality, his clown attire, and his infectious enthusiasm for bringing joy to others.

## 81. James Watson (USA) and Francis Crick (England): The Architects of DNA

- Opening Quote: "We have discovered the secret of life." - Francis Crick, upon realizing the structure of DNA.
- Historical Context: 1950s, the race to discover the structure of DNA, a competition that would revolutionize genetics and biology.
- Early Life & Influences: Watson, an American molecular biologist; Crick, a British physicist; they collaborated at the Cavendish Laboratory in Cambridge.
- Major Contributions:
  - Discovered the double helix structure of DNA in 1953: Built upon the work of Rosalind Franklin, Maurice Wilkins, and others.
- Challenges & Controversies: The limited recognition given to Rosalind Franklin for her critical contributions to the discovery, ethical questions about genetic engineering.
- Global Impact & Legacy:
  - Their discovery revolutionized biology and medicine, leading to advances in genetics, biotechnology, and personalized medicine.
  - Their work laid the foundation for the Human Genome Project and the emerging field of genomics.
- "Beyond the Scalpel": Watson and Crick's discovery is a testament to the power of collaboration, scientific curiosity, and the convergence of different fields of expertise.

## 82. Gro Harlem Brundtland (Norway): A Global Advocate for Health: From Public Health to Sustainable Development

- Opening Quote: "Health is a key indicator of sustainable development." – Gro Harlem Brundtland

- **Historical Context:** Late 20th and early 21st century, increasing recognition of the interconnectedness of health, environment, and development, the need for global cooperation to address health challenges.
- **Early Life & Influences:** Norwegian physician and politician, served as Prime Minister of Norway and as Director-General of the World Health Organization (WHO), a passionate advocate for global health and sustainable development.
- **Major Contributions:**
- **Chaired the World Commission on Environment and Development:** The commission's report, "Our Common Future" (1987), introduced the concept of sustainable development, emphasizing the interconnectedness of environmental, economic, and social issues, including health.
- **Led the WHO's Response to Global Health Challenges:** During her tenure as Director-General (1998-2003), she addressed issues such as HIV/AIDS, tuberculosis, malaria, and the emergence of new infectious diseases, advocating for increased funding, research, and access to healthcare.
- **Promoted the Social Determinants of Health:** Recognized the impact of social, economic, and environmental factors on health, advocating for policies to address these broader determinants and improve health equity.
- **Challenges & Controversies:** Navigating the political complexities of international health diplomacy, addressing the competing interests of different countries, and securing funding for global health initiatives.
- **Global Impact & Legacy:** Her leadership in global health and sustainable development has influenced policies and programs worldwide. Her work highlights the importance of a holistic and interdisciplinary approach to addressing health challenges and achieving health equity for all.
- **"Beyond the Scalpel":** Brundtland's career demonstrates the significant role that physicians can play in shaping public policy and advancing global health goals.

## 83. Elizabeth Kubler-Ross (Switzerland/USA): Pioneering Death and Dying

- Opening Quote: "The most beautiful people we have known are those who have known defeat, known suffering, known struggle, known loss, and have found their way out of the depths. These persons have an appreciation, sensitivity, and an understanding of life that fills them with compassions, gentleness, and a deep loving concern. Beautiful people do not just happen." - Elizabeth Kubler-Ross
- Historical Context: Mid-20th century, death and dying were taboo subjects, often hidden away from view, limited support for terminally ill patients and their families.

- Early Life & Influences: Swiss-American psychiatrist, deeply affected by her experiences working with terminally ill patients, challenged conventional approaches to death and dying.
- Major Contributions:
  - Wrote On Death and Dying (1969): Her groundbreaking work introduced the five stages of grief (denial, anger, bargaining, depression, acceptance).
  - Advocated for hospice care: Promoted a more humane and compassionate approach to end-of-life care, focusing on patient comfort and dignity.
- Challenges & Controversies: Her work on near-death experiences and the afterlife generated controversy, some critics questioned the validity of her five stages of grief model.
- Global Impact & Legacy:
  - Her work transformed the way we view and approach death and dying.
  - Her writings have helped millions of people cope with grief and loss.
- "Beyond the Scalpel": Kubler-Ross was a compassionate and empathetic individual, dedicated to bringing comfort and understanding to those facing death.

## 84. François Magendie (France): The Pioneer of Experimental Physiology

- Opening Quote: "Experiment is the only true guide in medical science." - François Magendie
- Historical Context: Early 19th century, physiology (the study of bodily functions) emerging as a distinct scientific discipline, a shift from observation to experimentation.
- Early Life & Influences: French physiologist, a strong advocate for the experimental method in medicine, challenged traditional medical thinking.
- Major Contributions:
  - Pioneered experimental physiology: Conducted numerous experiments on animals to understand the functions of the nervous system, digestion, and circulation.
  - Established the importance of control groups in experiments: A key principle of scientific research.
- Challenges & Controversies: His vivisection experiments on animals were criticized for their cruelty, raising ethical questions about animal experimentation in research.
- Global Impact & Legacy:
  - His work transformed the study of physiology, establishing the experimental method as the foundation for medical research.
  - His influence led to significant advances in understanding the human body and its functions.
- "Beyond the Scalpel": Magendie was known for his blunt and sometimes abrasive personality, but his dedication to scientific rigor and his commitment to advancing medical knowledge were undeniable.

## 85. William Stewart Halsted (USA): The Surgeon's Surgeon
- Opening Quote: "The surgeon must have an intuitive sense of the right thing to do." – William Stewart Halsted
- Historical Context: Late 19th and early 20th century, surgery was becoming more complex, the need for aseptic techniques, and the development of surgical residencies for training.
- Early Life & Influences: American surgeon, known for his meticulous surgical techniques and his contributions to surgical training, a complex figure who struggled with addiction but made significant contributions to medicine.
- Major Contributions:
    - Developed radical mastectomy for breast cancer: A controversial procedure, but it influenced surgical approaches to cancer treatment.
    - Introduced surgical gloves: To improve aseptic technique and reduce infection.
    - Established the first formal surgical residency program in the USA: At Johns Hopkins Hospital, his training model shaped surgical education.
- Challenges & Controversies: His addiction to cocaine and morphine, the long-term effects of radical mastectomy, the debate over his use of animal experimentation.
- Global Impact & Legacy:
    - His contributions to surgical techniques, aseptic practices, and surgical training have had a lasting impact on the field.
    - His legacy continues to inspire surgeons to strive for excellence and precision.
- "Beyond the Scalpel": Halsted's personal struggles with addiction highlight the pressures and complexities faced by medical professionals, even as they make significant contributions to their field.

## 86. Joseph Murray (USA): Transplantation Ethics and the Gift of Life
- Opening Quote: "The gift of life... is a gift that must be given freely and without any expectation of reward." – Joseph Murray
- Historical Context: Following the success of organ transplantation, the ethical considerations of organ allocation, donor consent, and the psychological impact of transplantation.
- Early Life & Influences: American surgeon, pioneer in organ transplantation, deeply concerned about the ethical and social implications of his work.
- Major Contributions:
    - Performed the first successful human kidney transplant in 1954: His work opened the door to organ transplantation as a life-saving treatment.

- - Wrote and lectured extensively on transplant ethics: Addressed issues of donor consent, organ allocation, and the psychological impact of transplantation.
- Challenges & Controversies: The ongoing shortage of organ donors, the high cost of transplant surgery, ethical concerns about the use of living donors.
- Global Impact & Legacy:
  - His pioneering work in transplantation led to the development of ethical guidelines and protocols.
  - His legacy continues to inspire efforts to improve organ donation rates and ensure equitable access to transplantation.
- "Beyond the Scalpel": Murray was a devout Catholic, his religious beliefs shaped his views on the sanctity of life and the importance of human dignity.

## 87. Audrey Evans (England/USA): The Angel of St. Jude

- Opening Quote: "Children are the future, and we must do everything we can to give them a chance to live." - Audrey Evans
- Historical Context: Mid-20th century, limited treatment options for childhood cancers, a lack of specialized pediatric cancer centers.
- Early Life & Influences: British-born American pediatric oncologist, dedicated to improving the care and treatment of children with cancer.
- Major Contributions:
  - Co-founded St. Jude Children's Research Hospital: A leading center for pediatric cancer research and treatment, providing free care to children with cancer.
  - Pioneered advancements in childhood leukemia treatment: Her work contributed to significant improvements in survival rates.
- Challenges & Controversies: The emotional toll of treating children with life-threatening illnesses, the ethical considerations of experimental cancer treatments.
- Global Impact & Legacy:
  - Her work has saved the lives of countless children with cancer.
  - St. Jude's research has led to advances in cancer treatment for children around the world.
- "Beyond the Scalpel": Evans was known for her compassion, her unwavering dedication to her patients, and her belief that every child deserves the chance to fight cancer.

## 88. William DeVries (USA): The Continuing Quest for the Artificial Heart

- Opening Quote: "The challenge of the artificial heart is not just to create a device that works, but to create a device that improves the quality of life." - William DeVries
- Historical Context: Following the first implant of a permanent artificial heart, the need to improve the technology and address the ethical and social implications.

- Early Life & Influences: American surgeon, a pioneer in artificial heart research and development, motivated by the desire to extend the lives of patients with end-stage heart failure.
- Major Contributions:
  - Continued to research and develop artificial heart technology: Worked on improving the design and functionality of artificial hearts, seeking to create a device that could provide long-term support.
  - Advocated for ethical guidelines: Addressed the complexities of artificial organ transplantation, including patient selection, quality of life, and the allocation of resources.
- Challenges & Controversies: The complexity and high cost of artificial heart technology, ethical debates about the definition of death and the appropriate use of artificial organs.
- Global Impact & Legacy:
  - His work advanced the field of artificial organ development, artificial hearts are now used as a bridge to transplantation and as a destination therapy for some patients.
  - His legacy continues to inspire research in bioengineering and the development of more advanced artificial organs.
- "Beyond the Scalpel": DeVries faced both celebration and criticism during his career, his work pushed the boundaries of medical technology and sparked ethical debates about the future of medicine.

## 89. Luc Montagnier (France): A Legacy of Scientific Inquiry and Controversy

- Opening Quote: "Science is not a dogma, it is a process of questioning and discovery." - Luc Montagnier
- Historical Context: Following the co-discovery of HIV, the ongoing research into HIV/AIDS treatment and prevention, the increasing scrutiny of scientific claims.
- Early Life & Influences: French virologist, known for his role in identifying HIV, continued to conduct research on various aspects of virology and immunology.
- Major Contributions:
  - Continued to research HIV/AIDS: Investigated potential cofactors in HIV infection, explored alternative treatment approaches.
- Challenges & Controversies: His later research on electromagnetic signals from DNA and his views on homeopathy generated skepticism and controversy within the scientific community.
- Global Impact & Legacy:
  - His work on HIV was critical in understanding the virus and developing treatments.
  - His later research remains controversial, highlighting the importance of scientific rigor and the need for evidence-based medicine.

- "Beyond the Scalpel": Montagnier's career exemplifies the complex relationship between scientific discovery, public perception, and the scrutiny of controversial research.

## 90. Anthony Fauci (USA): Guiding Public Health Policy

- Opening Quote: "You have to be very careful when you're dealing with a public health crisis... to make sure you don't overreact, but you also don't underreact." – Anthony Fauci
- Historical Context: Late 20th and early 21st century, the emergence of new infectious diseases (HIV/AIDS, Ebola, Zika, COVID-19), the need for effective public health leadership and communication.
- Early Life & Influences: American physician and immunologist, a leading expert on infectious diseases, dedicated to public service and science-based policymaking.
- Major Contributions:
    - Advised multiple presidential administrations: On HIV/AIDS, influenza, bioterrorism, and other public health threats.
    - Played a key role in shaping public health policy: Advocated for research funding, vaccine development, and public health education.
- Challenges & Controversies: Navigating the complex political landscape of public health, facing criticism for his handling of the COVID-19 pandemic.
- Global Impact & Legacy:
    - His leadership has guided public health policy in the U.S. and influenced global health efforts.
    - His advocacy for science and public health continues to be crucial in addressing emerging infectious diseases.
- "Beyond the Scalpel": Fauci is known for his tireless work ethic, his commitment to scientific integrity, and his ability to communicate complex medical information clearly to the public.

## 91. Jane Cooke Wright (USA): Breaking Barriers, Building a Legacy

- Opening Quote: [Find a quote that highlights Wright's commitment to mentoring and inspiring others.]
- Historical Context: Mid-20th century, the struggle for civil rights in the United States, limited opportunities for African Americans in medicine and science.
- Early Life & Influences: African American physician and researcher, a pioneer in cancer chemotherapy, dedicated to mentorship and improving cancer care for underserved communities.
- Major Contributions:
    - Mentored generations of medical students and researchers: Particularly encouraging African American women to pursue careers in medicine and science.
    - Advocated for health equity: Worked to improve access to cancer treatment for all patients, regardless of race or socioeconomic status.

- Challenges & Controversies: The persistent barriers of racial and gender discrimination, securing funding for research on cancer disparities.
- Global Impact & Legacy:
  - Her work in chemotherapy led to advancements in cancer treatment that have benefited patients worldwide.
  - Her legacy of mentorship and advocacy continues to inspire efforts to diversify the medical profession and address health disparities.
- "Beyond the Scalpel": Wright was a passionate advocate for education and believed that knowledge was the key to empowering individuals and communities.

## 92. Sir Frederick Gowland Hopkins (England): Unlocking the Mysteries of Vitamins

- Opening Quote: "Life is a dynamic equilibrium in a polyphasic system." – Frederick Gowland Hopkins
- Historical Context: Early 20th century, the emerging field of biochemistry, the discovery of "accessory food factors" (later known as vitamins) essential for health.
- Early Life & Influences: British biochemist, his research on nutrition and metabolism revolutionized the understanding of dietary essentials.
- Major Contributions:
- Discovered vitamins: His work established that vitamins are essential nutrients required for growth and health, deficiency diseases like scurvy and rickets could be prevented and treated with dietary supplements.
- Challenges & Controversies: The initial difficulty in isolating and identifying specific vitamins, the complex interplay of nutrients and their effects on health.
- Global Impact & Legacy:
- His work revolutionized the field of nutrition, leading to a better understanding of the role of vitamins in health and disease.
- His discoveries have had a major impact on public health, leading to the fortification of foods and the development of vitamin supplements to prevent deficiency diseases.
- "Beyond the Scalpel": Hopkins was a dedicated teacher and mentor, inspiring a generation of biochemists to explore the complexities of human metabolism and nutrition.
- 

## 93. James Barry (Ireland/England): The Surgeon Who Defied Gender Norms

- Opening Quote: [Omit a quote, as Barry's identity was a secret during their lifetime. Start with a statement about Barry's unconventional life and impact.]
- Historical Context: 19th century, rigid gender roles and societal expectations, women were largely excluded from medicine and the military.

- Early Life & Influences: Born Margaret Ann Bulkley in Ireland, lived as James Barry, a male military surgeon, their true identity was only revealed after death.
- Major Contributions:
  - Served as a military surgeon in the British Army: Posted to various locations, including South Africa and Canada, advocating for improved sanitation and healthcare for soldiers and the local population.
  - Performed the first successful caesarean section in Africa (1826): Saving the life of both the mother and child.
- Challenges & Controversies: Their true gender identity was a closely guarded secret, the social and personal implications of living as a man in a time when women were not permitted to practice medicine or serve in the military.
- Global Impact & Legacy:
  - Barry's story challenges our understanding of gender roles and identity, a remarkable example of overcoming societal barriers.
  - Their contributions to military medicine and public health demonstrate their commitment to serving others, regardless of personal risks.
- "Beyond the Scalpel": Barry's life was a testament to resilience and the pursuit of one's passion in the face of adversity.

## 94. Mary Putnam Jacobi (USA): Championing Women's Medical Education

- Opening Quote: "The only way to secure justice for women in medicine is to have women physicians." - Mary Putnam Jacobi
- Historical Context: Late 19th century, women were struggling to gain access to medical education and professional recognition, prevailing beliefs about women's intellectual capabilities limited their opportunities.
- Early Life & Influences: American physician and suffragist, a strong advocate for women's rights, particularly in medicine, her own experience navigating the male-dominated medical field shaped her advocacy.
- Major Contributions:
  - First woman admitted to the École de Médecine in Paris (1868): Faced resistance and discrimination, paving the way for other women.
  - Founded the Women's Medical College of the New York Infirmary: Providing quality medical education to women, contributing to the advancement of women in medicine.
- Challenges & Controversies: Persistent sexism in the medical field, challenges to women's scientific authority, the struggle for equal opportunities in research and practice.
- Global Impact & Legacy:
  - Her advocacy helped to open doors for women in medicine and other professions.

- - Her work on women's health and her contributions to medical education have had a lasting impact on healthcare.
  - "Beyond the Scalpel": Jacobi was also a prolific writer, publishing articles on medical topics, women's rights, and social issues, showcasing her intellectual versatility and commitment to progress.

## 95. David Baltimore (USA): Unlocking the Secrets of Retroviruses
- Opening Quote: "The greatest discoveries are often those we least expect." - David Baltimore
- Historical Context: 20th century, the emergence of molecular biology and the increasing understanding of viruses, particularly retroviruses like HIV.
- Early Life & Influences: American biologist, his research on retroviruses and reverse transcriptase revolutionized molecular biology and virology.
- Major Contributions:
  - Discovered reverse transcriptase: An enzyme that allows retroviruses to copy their RNA into DNA, a groundbreaking discovery with implications for understanding cancer and HIV.
- Challenges & Controversies: The complexities of retroviral research, the controversy surrounding accusations of scientific misconduct against a colleague, which tarnished his reputation.
- Global Impact & Legacy:
  - His work on reverse transcriptase was crucial to understanding how retroviruses function and replicate, leading to the development of antiretroviral drugs for HIV/AIDS.
  - His research continues to influence the development of gene therapy and other biotechnology applications.
- "Beyond the Scalpel": Baltimore has been a vocal advocate for science education and scientific integrity, emphasizing the importance of ethics in research.

## 96. Temple Grandin (USA): Understanding Autism and Animal Welfare
- Opening Quote: "The world needs all kinds of minds." - Temple Grandin
- Historical Context: 20th and 21st century, evolving understanding of autism and the need for humane treatment of animals in agriculture.
- Early Life & Influences: American scientist, animal behaviorist, and autism advocate, diagnosed with autism as a child, used her unique perspective to understand animal behavior and advocate for humane livestock handling.
- Major Contributions:
  - Revolutionized the livestock industry: Designed humane livestock handling facilities that reduce stress and improve animal welfare.

- o Wrote extensively about autism: Her books and lectures have helped to increase understanding and acceptance of people with autism.
- Challenges & Controversies: Overcoming the challenges of autism, advocating for animal welfare in an industry focused on efficiency, navigating the complexities of communicating her experiences and insights.
- Global Impact & Legacy:
  - o Her work has improved the lives of millions of animals in the livestock industry.
  - o Her writings and lectures have helped to reduce the stigma surrounding autism and promote inclusion.
- "Beyond the Scalpel": Grandin's story demonstrates the power of neurodiversity and the contributions that people with different ways of thinking can make to society.

## 97. Crawford Long (USA): The First to Use Ether Anesthesia

- Opening Quote: "Ether is inhaled until the patient becomes unconscious... then the operation is performed." - Crawford Long, describing his pioneering use of ether anesthesia.
- Historical Context: Early 19th century, surgery was excruciatingly painful, limiting the types of procedures that could be performed.
- Early Life & Influences: American physician and pharmacist, interested in the effects of nitrous oxide (laughing gas), discovered the anesthetic properties of ether.
- Major Contributions:
  - o First to use ether anesthesia during surgery (1842): His discovery revolutionized surgery by making painless operations possible.
- Challenges & Controversies: He did not publish his findings immediately, delaying wider recognition of his discovery, leading to disputes about who should receive credit for pioneering ether anesthesia.
- Global Impact & Legacy:
  - o His discovery transformed surgical practice, allowing for more complex and lengthy procedures, and dramatically reducing patient suffering.
  - o His work paved the way for the development of modern anesthesiology and the use of various anesthetic agents.
- "Beyond the Scalpel": Long was a quiet and unassuming individual who prioritized his patients' well-being, his reluctance to promote his own discovery reflects his humble nature.

## 98. Surgeon General C. Everett Koop (USA): Public Health Advocacy in the Face of Controversy

- Opening Quote: "The only safe sex is abstinence." – C. Everett Koop, a statement that reflects his controversial views on HIV/AIDS prevention.
- Historical Context: 1980s, the HIV/AIDS epidemic was emerging, political and social controversies surrounding public health measures.

- Early Life & Influences: American pediatric surgeon, appointed Surgeon General by President Ronald Reagan, known for his strong conservative views, surprised many by his frank approach to HIV/AIDS education.
- Major Contributions:
  - Published a groundbreaking report on HIV/AIDS: (1986) Advocated for public education about HIV transmission and prevention, challenged the stigma surrounding the disease.
  - Promoted public health measures: Campaigned against smoking, advocated for seat belt use, addressed issues of drug abuse and violence.
- Challenges & Controversies: His conservative views clashed with public health approaches to HIV/AIDS prevention, faced criticism from both conservatives and liberals.
- Global Impact & Legacy:
  - His work helped to raise awareness about HIV/AIDS and reduce the stigma associated with the disease.
  - His example highlighted the role of the Surgeon General in providing evidence-based public health information, even in the face of political pressures.
- "Beyond the Scalpel": Koop was a devout Christian, his faith informed his views on healthcare and bioethics.

## 99. Harold Freeman (USA): Champion of Cancer Care Equity

- Opening Quote: "Healthcare is a right, not a privilege." – Harold Freeman, summarizing his life's work.
- Historical Context: Late 20th and early 21st century, growing recognition of racial disparities in cancer care and outcomes, the need for systemic change to ensure health equity.
- Early Life & Influences: African American surgeon and oncologist, a leading advocate for eliminating disparities in cancer care, dedicated to improving access to cancer screening and treatment for underserved communities.
- Major Contributions:
  - Founded the Ralph Lauren Center for Cancer Care and Prevention in Harlem: A model for providing quality cancer care in underserved communities.
  - Developed the "Patient Navigation" model: Assisting patients in navigating the complex healthcare system, improving access to timely diagnosis and treatment.
- Challenges & Controversies: The persistent and systemic nature of racial disparities in healthcare, securing funding for programs to address healthcare inequities.
- Global Impact & Legacy:
  - His work has helped to reduce disparities in cancer care and improve outcomes for minority patients.
  - His legacy continues to inspire efforts to achieve health equity for all.

- "Beyond the Scalpel": Freeman was a compassionate and dedicated physician, known for his commitment to his patients and his unwavering belief that all people deserve quality healthcare.

## 100. Atul Gawande (USA): Rethinking Modern Medicine

- Opening Quote: "Better is possible. It does not take genius. It takes diligence. It takes moral clarity. It takes ingenuity. And above all, it takes a willingness to try." – Atul Gawande
- Historical Context: 21st century, the complexities of modern medicine, the rising costs of healthcare, the need for a more humane and patient-centered approach.
- Early Life & Influences: American surgeon and writer, his books and articles have explored the challenges and possibilities of modern medicine, advocating for improvements in healthcare delivery and patient experience.
- Major Contributions:
    - Wrote bestselling books: Complications, Better, The Checklist Manifesto, and Being Mortal, examining the human side of medicine, the importance of communication, and the challenges of aging and death.
    - Founded Ariadne Labs: A research and innovation center focused on improving healthcare delivery, particularly in the areas of surgery, childbirth, and end-of-life care.
- Challenges & Controversies: The complexities of healthcare reform, addressing the financial incentives in healthcare, the tension between technology and humanism in medicine.
- Global Impact & Legacy:
    - His writing has sparked conversations about the future of healthcare and the importance of patient-centered care.
    - His work has led to practical improvements in healthcare delivery, particularly through the use of checklists and other strategies to reduce errors.
- "Beyond the Scalpel": Gawande is known for his thoughtful and engaging writing style, his ability to connect with both medical professionals and the general public, sparking reflection and discussion about the human experience of illness and healthcare.

# Conclusion

As we conclude this journey through the lives of 100 remarkable healers, scientists, and innovators, we stand in awe of the human capacity to alleviate suffering and to push the boundaries of medical knowledge. From ancient practices to cutting-edge technologies, the story of medicine is a testament to our collective quest for a healthier future.

Throughout these narratives, several enduring themes have emerged. We have witnessed the power of **keen observation** – exemplified by Hippocrates, who urged physicians to "examine for the most minute signs," and by John Snow, who meticulously mapped a cholera outbreak to identify its source. We have marveled at the courage to **challenge dogma** – seen in Ignaz Semmelweis's relentless campaign for hand hygiene despite opposition from the medical establishment, and Elizabeth Kenny's unorthodox approach to polio treatment. We have been inspired by the **spirit of innovation** – from Ambroise Paré's gentler surgical techniques to Christiaan Barnard's groundbreaking heart transplant.

Yet, the history of medicine is not without its shadows. We have also confronted the ethical dilemmas that arise when pushing the boundaries of knowledge – as in the case of Aubrey Levin, whose abuse of power serves as a stark reminder of the responsibility that comes with the healing profession. And we have seen how prejudice and discrimination have often hindered progress and excluded brilliant minds, as exemplified by the struggles of countless women and individuals from marginalized communities.

As we look to the future of medicine, the lessons learned from these trailblazers become ever more important. We face new challenges – from emerging infectious diseases to the complexities of an aging population, from the ethical questions surrounding genetic manipulation to the disparities in healthcare access around the world.

Yet, the spirit of those who came before us provides a guiding light. They remind us to:

- **Embrace the Power of Observation:** To see the details, question assumptions, and constantly seek a deeper understanding of the human body and disease.

- **Foster Innovation, But Proceed with Caution:** To push the boundaries of knowledge, but with a deep sense of ethical responsibility and respect for the dignity of every patient.
- **Champion Collaboration:** To break down silos, work across disciplines, and recognize that progress often emerges from the convergence of diverse perspectives and expertise.
- **Advocate for Equity and Access:** To ensure that the benefits of medical advancements reach all members of society, regardless of background or circumstance.

The journey of medicine is an unfinished one. The 100 individuals highlighted in this book represent a fraction of the countless individuals who have contributed to the advancement of human health. Their stories serve as a reminder that every physician, nurse, scientist, and advocate has the potential to make a difference. By embracing the legacy of those who came before us and carrying forward the torch of medical progress, we can shape a future where healthcare is truly accessible, equitable, and transformative for all.

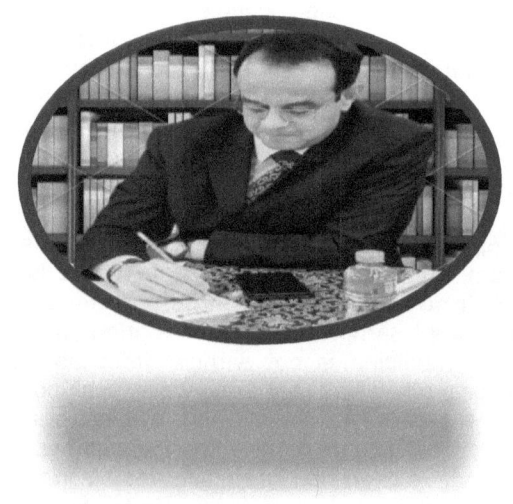

*Dr. Atef Ahmed*

[2024]

books.dratef.net

dratef1980@gmail.com

# References

1. Majno, G. (1975). *The Healing Hand: Man and Wound in the Ancient World*. Harvard University Press.
2. Das, G. (2013). *The Surgery of Sushruta*. Motilal Banarsidass.
3. Farmer, P. (2003). *Pathologies of Power: Health, Human Rights, and the New War on the Poor*. University of California Press.
4. Goldstein, J. (2004). *Avicenna and the Visionary Recital*. Cambridge University Press.
5. Grandin, T. (2005). *Animals in Translation: Using the Mysteries of Autism to Decode Animal Behavior*. Scribner.
6. Collins, F. S. (2006). *The Language of God: A Scientist Presents Evidence for Belief*. Free Press.
7. Porter, R. (Ed.). (2006). *The Cambridge Illustrated History of Medicine*. Cambridge University Press.
8. McDougall, R. (2007). *The Killing of a Cure: The Campaign to Combat Polio*. University of Queensland Press.
9. Bynum, W.F., & Porter, R. (Eds.). (2009). *Companion Encyclopedia of the History of Medicine*. Routledge.
10. Lock, S., Reynolds, A., & Tansey, E. M. (Eds.). (2009). *The Oxford Illustrated Companion to Medicine*. Oxford University Press.
11. Mukherjee, S. (2010). *The Emperor of All Maladies: A Biography of Cancer*. Scribner.
12. Duffin, J. (2010). *History of Medicine: A Scandalously Short Introduction*. University of Toronto Press.
13. Janzen, J. M., & Feierman, S. (Eds.). (2013). *The Social History of Health and Medicine in Africa*. Palgrave Macmillan.
14. Hajar, R. (2013). *The History of Cardiology*. Elsevier.
15. Gawande, A. (2014). *Being Mortal: Medicine and What Matters in the End*. Metropolitan Books.
16. Conrad, L. I., Neve, M., Nutton, V., Porter, R., & Wear, A. (Eds.). (2016). *The Western Medical Tradition: 800 BCE to 1800 CE*. Cambridge University Press.
17. Fitzharris, L. (2017). *The Butchering Art: Joseph Lister's Quest to Transform the Grisly World of Victorian Medicine*. Scientific American/Farrar, Straus and Giroux.

18. Nuland, S. B. (1988). *Doctors: The Biography of Medicine*. Alfred A. Knopf.
19. Gay, P. (1988). *Freud: A Life for Our Time*. W. W. Norton & Company.
20. Porter, R. (1997). *The Greatest Benefit to Mankind: A Medical History of Humanity from Antiquity to the Present*. W. W. Norton & Company.

# Index

1. **Hippocrates (Ancient Greece):** The Father of Western Medicine, known for the Hippocratic Oath and emphasis on clinical observation.
2. **Sushruta (Ancient India):** The Father of Surgery in Ayurveda, author of the *Sushruta Samhita*, detailing surgical techniques and instruments.
3. **Zhang Zhongjing (Ancient China):** The Sage of Traditional Chinese Medicine, author of *Shang Han Lun*, foundational text on Cold Damage disorders.
4. **Agnodice (Ancient Greece):** Legendary female physician who challenged gender barriers in ancient Greece by disguising herself as a man to practice medicine.
5. **Pedanius Dioscorides (Ancient Rome):** Author of *De Materia Medica*, a comprehensive encyclopedia of medicinal plants that influenced pharmacology for centuries.
6. **Galen (Ancient Rome):** Prolific writer on medicine and anatomy, influential for over 1,500 years, known for his theory of the four humors.
7. **Al-Razi (Rhazes) (Persia):** Clinician and empiricist, author of *Al-Hawi (The Comprehensive Book)*, known for differentiating smallpox from measles.
8. **Avicenna (Ibn Sina) (Persia):** Polymath physician, author of *The Canon of Medicine*, synthesized medical knowledge from East and West, introduced new ideas such as quarantine.
9. **Trotula of Salerno (Italy):** Medieval woman physician, associated with the *Trotula*, a collection of texts on women's health, demonstrating the vital role of women in healthcare history.
10. **Ibn al-Nafis (Syria):** Anatomist who corrected Galen's errors, providing the first accurate description of pulmonary circulation, highlighting advancements in Islamic medicine.
11. **Hildegard von Bingen (Germany):** Benedictine abbess, visionary, and healer, wrote on natural history and medicine, advocating a holistic approach to health and well-being.
12. **Andreas Vesalius (Flanders):** Revolutionized anatomy with his groundbreaking work *De Humani Corporis Fabrica*, featuring detailed illustrations based on his dissections.
13. **Ambroise Paré (France):** Father of modern surgery, known for rejecting cauterization of wounds and introducing gentler surgical techniques, also improved prosthetics.
14. **William Harvey (England):** Discovered the circulation of blood, publishing *De Motu Cordis*, detailing his experiments and observations.
15. **Paracelsus (Switzerland):** Alchemist physician who challenged traditional medical authority, introduced the use of chemicals in medicine, and advocated for observation and experimentation.
16. **Edward Jenner (England):** Pioneer of vaccination, developed the smallpox vaccine, leading to the eventual eradication of this deadly disease.
17. **James Parkinson (England):** Identified Parkinson's disease, meticulously describing its symptoms in his essay *An Essay on the Shaking Palsy*.
18. **René Laennec (France):** Inventor of the stethoscope, revolutionizing medical diagnosis by allowing doctors to hear heart and lung sounds clearly.
19. **Ignaz Semmelweis (Hungary):** Discoverer of the link between hand hygiene and puerperal fever, champion of antiseptic practices that saved countless lives.
20. **Florence Nightingale (England):** Founder of modern nursing, known for her contributions to sanitation and hospital reform during the Crimean War, established professional nursing schools.
21. **Elizabeth Blackwell (USA):** The first woman to receive a medical degree in the United States, founded hospitals for women and children, and a tireless advocate for women in medicine.
22. **Louis Pasteur (France):** The Father of Microbiology, developed germ theory, pasteurization, and vaccines for rabies, anthrax, and chicken cholera.
23. **Robert Koch (Germany):** The Father of Bacteriology, identified the bacteria causing anthrax, tuberculosis, and cholera, established Koch's Postulates, foundational to modern microbiology.
24. **Joseph Lister (England):** Pioneer of antiseptic surgery, introduced carbolic acid for sterilization, dramatically reducing postoperative infection rates.
25. **Marie Curie (Poland/France):** Pioneer in the study of radioactivity, discovered polonium and radium, developed techniques for isolating radioactive isotopes, the first woman to win a Nobel Prize and the only person to win in two different scientific fields.
26. **Sigmund Freud (Austria):** The Father of Psychoanalysis, developed psychoanalysis as a theory of the mind and a method of treatment for mental illness.

27. **Alexander Fleming (Scotland):** Discoverer of penicillin, the first antibiotic, his serendipitous finding revolutionized the treatment of bacterial infections.
28. **Frederick Banting (Canada):** Co-discoverer of insulin, along with Charles Best, transformed the treatment of diabetes from a fatal disease to a manageable condition.
29. **Virginia Apgar (USA):** Developed the Apgar Score, a simple but effective method for assessing newborn health, revolutionizing neonatal care.
30. **Jonas Salk (USA):** Developer of the inactivated polio vaccine (IPV), a major breakthrough in the fight against polio.
31. **Helen Brooke Taussig (USA):** Pioneer in pediatric cardiology, instrumental in developing the Blalock-Taussig shunt for "blue babies" (infants with cyanotic heart disease).
32. **Christiaan Barnard (South Africa):** Performed the world's first successful human-to-human heart transplant, raising the profile of transplant surgery and igniting ethical debate.
33. **Norman Shumway (USA):** Pioneer of heart-lung transplantation, advanced the field of transplantation, opening new possibilities for treating complex heart and lung conditions.
34. **Tu Youyou (China):** Discovered artemisinin, a powerful antimalarial drug derived from the sweet wormwood plant, a traditional Chinese remedy, demonstrating the value of exploring traditional medicine for new drug discoveries.
35. **David Ho (Taiwan/USA):** Pioneer of HIV/AIDS research, developed combination antiretroviral therapy (ART), dramatically improving the lives of people living with HIV/AIDS.
36. **Paul Farmer (USA):** Champion of global health equity, co-founded Partners In Health (PIH), providing healthcare to the poor, and advocate for social justice and addressing the social determinants of health.
37. **Ben Carson (USA):** Renowned pediatric neurosurgeon, pioneer of hemispherectomy for severe epilepsy, known for his successful separation of conjoined twins.
38. **Elizabeth Garrett Anderson (England):** First woman to qualify as a physician and surgeon in Britain, established a hospital for women staffed entirely by women, and a prominent advocate for women's suffrage.
39. **Wilhelm Conrad Röntgen (Germany):** Discoverer of X-rays, revolutionized medical diagnostics, making it possible to see inside the human body without surgery.
40. **Sir William Osler (Canada):** Considered the "Father of Modern Medicine," known for his influential textbook *The Principles and Practice of Medicine*, his emphasis on bedside teaching, and his humanistic approach to medicine.
41. **Karl Landsteiner (Austria):** Discoverer of the ABO blood groups, his work made safe blood transfusions possible and revolutionized the field of hematology.
42. **Harvey Cushing (USA):** The Father of Neurosurgery, known for his pioneering techniques, his meticulous approach to brain surgery, and his contributions to the understanding and treatment of brain tumors.
43. **Howard Florey (Australia) and Ernst Boris Chain (Germany):** Key figures in the development of penicillin as a practical therapeutic drug, their work made penicillin widely available, saving countless lives, particularly during World War II.
44. **Selman Waksman (Ukraine/USA):** Discoverer of streptomycin, the first effective antibiotic for tuberculosis, a pioneer in soil microbiology research.
45. **Albert Sabin (Poland/USA):** Developer of the oral polio vaccine (OPV), using a live, weakened virus, played a crucial role in global efforts to eradicate polio.
46. **Gertrude B. Elion (USA):** Pioneer in drug development and rational drug design, developed numerous drugs for leukemia, malaria, gout, herpes, and organ transplant rejection, her work significantly advanced the field of pharmacology.
47. **Margaret Sanger (USA):** Controversial advocate for women's reproductive rights, founded the organization that would become Planned Parenthood, fought for access to birth control information and services.
48. **Hua Tuo (Ancient China):** Renowned surgeon and physician of the Han Dynasty, credited with developing a form of surgical anesthesia, advocated for physical exercise and therapeutic movement.
49. **Michael DeBakey (USA):** A master of cardiovascular surgery, pioneered techniques for repairing aortic aneurysms, performed early coronary artery bypass surgeries, developed the MASH unit concept, and was influential in medical diplomacy.
50. **C. Walton Lillehei (USA):** A pioneer of open-heart surgery, developed the cross-circulation technique and helped develop the heart-lung machine, making open-heart surgery possible, a dedicated teacher who mentored generations of surgeons.
51. **Harold Gillies (New Zealand/England):** The Father of Plastic Surgery, developed innovative techniques for reconstructive surgery during World War I, established a dedicated plastic surgery hospital, and founded the British Association of Plastic Surgeons.
52. **Willem Johan Kolff (Netherlands/USA):** A visionary in the field of artificial organs, developed the first working artificial kidney (hemodialysis machine) and the first artificial heart, his work transformed the treatment of kidney failure and inspired research on other artificial organs.
53. **Charles Richard Drew (USA):** Pioneer of blood banking, developed methods for blood storage and preservation, directed the blood plasma program during World War II, and challenged racial segregation in blood donation, advocating for equality in healthcare.
54. **Alfred Blalock (USA) & Vivien Thomas (USA):** A collaborative surgical duo who developed the Blalock-Taussig shunt, a groundbreaking procedure that saved the lives of countless children with "blue baby syndrome," their story highlights the importance of collaboration and overcoming racial barriers in medicine.
55. **Jonas Edward Salk (USA):** Developer of the inactivated polio vaccine (IPV), his work had a major impact on public health and the near-eradication of polio, also a thoughtful writer on biophilosophy, exploring the ethical implications of science.

56. **Godfrey Hounsfield (England):** Developed the computed tomography (CT) scanner, a revolutionary medical imaging technology that provides detailed cross-sectional images of the body, transforming the diagnosis and treatment of various diseases.
57. **Aubrey Levin (South Africa/Canada):** Psychiatrist, his career ended in disgrace due to his conviction for sexual assault of patients, a cautionary tale about abuse of power and the importance of medical ethics.
58. **William DeVries (USA):** A pioneer in artificial heart research, implanted the first permanent artificial heart (Jarvik-7), advancing artificial organ development and raising ethical questions about life-extending technologies.
59. **Robert Gallo (USA):** Co-discoverer of the human immunodeficiency virus (HIV), played a critical role in understanding the cause of AIDS, his work led to the development of HIV blood tests and treatments.
60. **Luc Montagnier (France):** Co-discoverer of HIV, led the team that first identified the virus, his later research on electromagnetic signals from DNA sparked controversy.
61. **Anthony Fauci (USA):** A leading expert on infectious diseases, served as a trusted advisor to multiple U.S. presidents, guided public health policy, and played a key role in the response to major outbreaks, including HIV/AIDS and COVID-19.
62. **Jane Cooke Wright (USA):** A pioneer in cancer chemotherapy, developed new treatments, particularly for leukemia, broke racial and gender barriers in medicine, and served as a role model for aspiring physicians, especially African American women.
63. **Harold Varmus (USA):** Nobel laureate for his research on oncogenes (genes that can cause cancer), served as director of the National Institutes of Health (NIH) and the National Cancer Institute (NCI), and a strong advocate for open access to scientific research.
64. **Elizabeth Kenny (Australia):** Developed the "Kenny Method" for treating polio, emphasizing muscle re-education and exercise over immobilization, challenged conventional medical wisdom, and transformed the field of physical therapy.
65. **Harold Freeman (USA):** A champion of cancer care equity, founded the Ralph Lauren Center for Cancer Care and Prevention in Harlem, developed the "Patient Navigation" model to guide underserved patients through the healthcare system.
66. **Helen Taussig (USA):** Founder of pediatric cardiology, dedicated her life to improving the lives of children with heart defects, instrumental in developing the Blalock-Taussig shunt for "blue babies," a pioneer for women in medicine.
67. **Al-Zahrawi (Abulcasis) (Islamic Spain):** A renowned surgeon of the Islamic Golden Age, his medical encyclopedia, *Al-Tasrif*, was influential in Europe for centuries, considered the father of modern surgery in the West.
68. **Jean-Martin Charcot (France):** Considered the father of modern neurology, systematically studied neurological disorders, his descriptions and classifications of diseases like multiple sclerosis and ALS are still used today.
69. **C. Walton Lillehei (USA):** A pioneer of open-heart surgery, known for developing techniques that made open-heart surgery possible, a gifted teacher and mentor who trained generations of cardiac surgeons.
70. **Harold Gillies (New Zealand/England):** A pioneer of plastic surgery, developed innovative reconstructive techniques during World War I, established a dedicated plastic surgery hospital, and advanced the field of plastic and reconstructive surgery.
71. **Willem Johan Kolff (Netherlands/USA):** A visionary inventor, developed the first working artificial kidney (hemodialysis machine) and artificial heart, his work revolutionized the treatment of kidney failure and inspired the field of bioengineering.
72. **Charles Richard Drew (USA):** Pioneer of blood banking, developed methods for blood storage and preservation, challenged racial segregation in blood donation, his work has had a lasting impact on blood transfusion safety and equity.
73. **Alfred Blalock (USA):** A skilled cardiac surgeon known for his bold approaches, challenged racial barriers in medicine by working closely with Vivien Thomas, an African American surgical technician, their partnership resulted in the life-saving Blalock-Taussig shunt.
74. **Selman Waksman (Ukraine/USA):** A pioneer in the field of soil microbiology, he discovered streptomycin and other antibiotics, his research has saved countless lives and advanced the development of new antibiotics.
75. **Albert Sabin (Poland/USA):** Developed the oral polio vaccine (OPV) using a live, attenuated virus, his vaccine played a crucial role in global polio eradication efforts.
76. **Gertrude B. Elion (USA):** A pioneer in rational drug design, developed numerous drugs for leukemia, malaria, herpes, and organ transplant rejection, her work revolutionized drug development and led to significant improvements in the treatment of various diseases.
77. **Denton Cooley (USA):** A giant in cardiac surgery, known for performing the first successful implantation of a total artificial heart in the United States, also developed techniques for repairing aortic aneurysms.
78. **Imhotep (Ancient Egypt):** An ancient Egyptian polymath, revered as a god of healing and wisdom, credited with medical texts and architectural achievements, his legacy highlights the interconnectedness of medicine and spirituality.
79. **Thomas Starzl (USA):** The Father of Modern Transplantation, performed the first successful human liver transplant, and developed immunosuppressive regimens, his work transformed the field of organ transplantation and saved countless lives.
80. **Patch Adams (USA):** A physician, social activist, and founder of the Gesundheit! Institute, he promoted the therapeutic value of laughter and advocated for holistic and compassionate care in medicine.
81. **James Watson (USA) & Francis Crick (England):** Co-discoverers of the double helix structure of DNA, their work revolutionized biology and medicine, paving the way for advances in genetics, biotechnology, and personalized medicine.

82. **Gro Harlem Brundtland (Norway):** A physician and politician, she served as Prime Minister of Norway and Director-General of the World Health Organization (WHO), advocating for global health equity, sustainable development, and addressing the social determinants of health.
83. **Elisabeth Kübler-Ross (Switzerland/USA):** A psychiatrist who transformed our understanding of death and dying, she introduced the five stages of grief and advocated for hospice care, promoting a more humane approach to end-of-life care.
84. **François Magendie (France):** A pioneer in experimental physiology, he emphasized the importance of the experimental method in medicine, conducting numerous experiments to understand the nervous system, digestion, and circulation.
85. **William Stewart Halsted (USA):** Considered the "Father of Modern Surgery," he was a skilled surgeon who developed innovative techniques, introduced surgical gloves, and established the first formal surgical residency program in the United States.
86. **Joseph Murray (USA):** Pioneer in organ transplantation, he performed the first successful human kidney transplant, opening the door to organ transplantation as a life-saving treatment, also explored the ethical aspects of transplantation.
87. **Audrey Evans (England/USA):** A pediatric oncologist dedicated to improving the lives of children with cancer, co-founded St. Jude Children's Research Hospital, and pioneered advancements in childhood leukemia treatment.
88. **William DeVries (USA):** A pioneer in artificial heart research, he implanted the first permanent artificial heart, advancing the field of artificial organs and raising ethical questions about life-extending technology.
89. **Luc Montagnier (France):** A virologist who co-discovered HIV, his work was crucial in understanding the virus and developing treatments, his later research on electromagnetic signals from DNA was controversial.
90. **Anthony Fauci (USA):** A leading figure in infectious disease research and public health, he has served as a key advisor to multiple U.S. presidents and has played a crucial role in shaping the response to major outbreaks, including HIV/AIDS and COVID-19.
91. **Jane Cooke Wright (USA):** A pioneer in chemotherapy research, especially for leukemia, she broke racial and gender barriers in medicine, becoming a role model for aspiring African American women in science and medicine.
92. **Sir Frederick Gowland Hopkins (England):** A Nobel laureate in Physiology or Medicine, he is considered one of the founders of biochemistry, known for his discovery of vitamins and their importance to human health.
93. **James Barry (Ireland/England):** A military surgeon who served in the British Army while concealing their female identity, their story challenges our understanding of gender roles and highlights the barriers women faced in medicine and the military during the 19th century.
94. **Mary Putnam Jacobi (USA):** A physician and suffragist who fought for women's rights in medicine, she was the first woman admitted to the École de Médecine in Paris and co-founded the Women's Medical College of the New York Infirmary.
95. **David Baltimore (USA):** A Nobel laureate in Physiology or Medicine for his discovery of reverse transcriptase, an enzyme that plays a key role in retroviruses like HIV, his work has had a significant impact on the development of antiretroviral drugs for HIV/AIDS.
96. **Temple Grandin (USA):** A professor of animal science, autism advocate, and author, she revolutionized the livestock industry by designing humane animal handling facilities, her work has improved animal welfare and fostered a better understanding of autism.
97. **Crawford Long (USA):** A pioneer in anesthesiology, he was the first to use ether as an anesthetic during surgery, his discovery revolutionized surgical practice, making it possible to perform painless operations.
98. **C. Everett Koop (USA):** Surgeon General of the United States, known for his frank and controversial report on HIV/AIDS in 1986, which advocated for public education about the disease and challenged the stigma surrounding it.
99. **Harold Freeman (USA):** A champion of cancer care equity, he dedicated his career to improving access to cancer treatment for underserved communities and developed the "Patient Navigation" model to help patients navigate the healthcare system.
100. **Atul Gawande (USA):** A surgeon and prolific writer, he has explored the complexities of modern medicine, advocated for patient-centered care, and sparked important conversations about healthcare delivery, surgical safety, and end-of-life care.

# Author's Profile

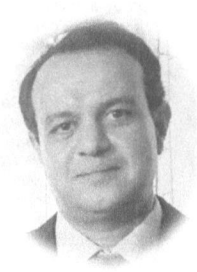

Name: Atef Ahmed Abdelrahim
Date of Birth: June 1978
Zodiac Sign: Cancer
Place of Birth: Asyut Governorate, Arab Republic of Egypt
Education:
Graduate of the Faculty of Medicine, Asyut University
Passionate about medical and literary research
Avid reader since childhood
Consultant Surgeon in the Arab Republic of Egypt
Has diverse experiences in various fields, including:

- Web development

- Android application programming

- Video content creation on YouTube Has authored numerous works in literature, personal development, and medicine Proficient in multiple languages, including published works and works in progress.

books.dratef.net
dratef1980@gmail.com

All Copywright Preserved to

Atef Ahmed Abd El Raheem
2024
ISBN: 9798334899087
Imprint: Independently published

www.ingramcontent.com/pod-product-compliance
Lightning Source LLC
Chambersburg PA
CBHW030503220526
45464CB00006B/2635